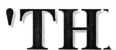 

Anybody Can Learn to Become Telekinetic & Master the Secrets of True Psychokinesis.

by

Gita Sudarshanananda

ISBN: 978-0-615-23737-4

www.thisispk.org

Table of Contents

Introduction:

"One who has experienced his own true identity understands that all things exist as paraphernalia for giving ecstatic pleasure to the Supreme Lord."

(Srila Bhaktisiddhanta Sarasvati Thakura - Commentary on Srimad-Bhagavatam 11.2.41)

The underlying purpose of this book is to educate readers about important discoveries that the author has made in the fields of psychokinesis, mind over matter and metaphysics. This manuscript is also designed to show readers that transcendental yoga and meditation (TM) were the keys to author's most magnificent discovery known as the Fridge Phenomenon (FP). For me, these breakthroughs substantiate the power of metaphysical and spiritual practices including disciplinary yoga. Here, you are generously given the secrets for understanding and developing real telekinetic powers. Readers are provided the same tools that the author personally uses to control the principle of psychokinesis (PK).

This book specifically educates readers about how powerful mind over matter forces can indeed be controlled. Knowledge is useless with out methods, systems, techniques and processes for applying it towards definite ends. So, this handbook shows readers exactly how to apply this highly specialized transcendental knowledge to the fabric of life itself. The secret to life is learning to control it as much as possible, and this manuscript certainly makes that possible for readers. The rigid and useless ways of thinking that many have grown accustomed to are now breaking down and being supplanted by the "Absolute Truth!" This concrete truth is all that can set us free, and lead our minds to the plane of liberation or nirvana.

Everything in our human existence is a product of mind over matter either at some level. It is a power that lies within everybody but they must learn to use it otherwise it's virtually useless. We have been mentally controlling the physical plane, either consciously or unconsciously, since the day we were born. From the start of life, all of our minds have varying degrees of control over matter, in accordance with the complexities of our karmas, chakra dispositions, and individual uniqueness. This book gives you the keys, knowledge, mystical tools and secrets to understanding and control the principle of mind over matter. It proves to readers how the mind can directly control physical objects, events, and even people in our environment! Just like driving a car, with a little practice, persistence, and perseverance, you can have the control over life that you have always dreamed of. Since the remotest of recorded times on Earth, man has been quite aware of the mental basis of reality. This book is a resource that presents secret knowledge regarding PK that most people in society have easily overlooked, due to the highly advanced and specialized nature of the formal research. This teaches readers how to develop their own selves to the fullest, by applying that very same knowledge directly to our most important energy centers.

In reality, paranormal experiences are an indispensable part of spiritual enlightenment. I only was fortunate enough to make my main discovery in PK (the FP) because of stumbling on sacred transcendental information that only the best of Karma can bring. In this book you will read about how this all resonated into me proving mind over matter scientifically. Like anybody who discovers a new resource or phenomenon, I know more about it then others who are mere observers studying things from the outside looking in. By analogy, Einstein made his discoveries only because he knew far more about physics that other people. So you can obviously learn a great deal from people who make valid discoveries and we are the best Gurus.

In all cultures throughout history, there are reports where objects or events in the environment are apparently influenced human minds. Do certain people actually have telekinetic or electrokinetic powers? Do you possess these superhuman abilities and if so, to what degree? Can this energy be triggered, amplified, and directed to act upon our lives in useful ways? What are the direct correlations between the practice of mystical yoga and   PK mind over matter?

This manuscript explores these issues in-depth, enabling readers to draw their own inferences concerning the bourgeoning science of mind over matter. Do yourself a favor and discard any presuppositions about this subject matter. Open your mind up to a whole new higher dimension of possibilities for all. The Fridge Phenomenon (FP) is a newly discovered manifestation of True-PK that gave rise to this entire book! True PK can be sharply distinguished from other so-called psychokinetic effects designed to fool the masses. In the case of true PK, no physical contact whatsoever is involved with the object being effected by the mind.

In True PK, there is basically no way, under conventional scientific thought, of explaining how the mind remotely controls physical objects and events. True PK involves no trickery or sleight of hand. Examples may include materialization phenomenon, bilocation, levitation, weather control, influencing the physical whereabouts of others, and effecting objects at any distance. It also involves the ability to directly influence the behavior of subatomic particles at the "quantum level."

This handbook proves to you that the existence of PK force and mind over matter is a "matter of fact." It is unequivocally proven consistently through the FP and many other telekinetic effects. You will study and learn how PK works; that it is indeed a very real and objective source of energy just like any other. The fact that PK exists and can directly control matter is old news for people like myself, and all who are intelligent enough to understand the nature and reality of the FP. PK is a force that can be directly monitored and influenced by certain mental techniques and technologies.

Contrary to what some people think, PK force is not a matter of occult pop-fiction or mere fantasy. It is a very real force that can apparently make anything happen for you if used properly and mastered. The good news is that this force and the principles for controlling it are not so difficult to learn; and the secrets are in your hands. The not so good news is that if people do not learn how it works, life itself can be placed at great jeopardy depending on one's karma.

Practicing distinct forms of transcendental meditation and yoga have always been powerful ways of boosting the mental capabilities. Naturally, everybody loves to hear or read about the transcendental glories and pastimes of Lord Krsna, as they put the mind at ease. That is because we all have an eternal relationship with Him. And, by restoring that eternal relationship with knowledge and intelligence, we are situated back on our constitutional positions as divine cosmic beings! To some degree, we have all been attenuated from the spiritual world which is our real home. Being disconnected from that world is the main cause of unhappiness, anxiety and discontent in our world.

Transcendental knowledge such as the pastimes of Lord Sri Krsna tunes our minds back into the spiritual world and all of its celestial energies. The author maintains that meditating on the transcendental glories and pastimes of Lord Krsna is indeed the most powerful way of creating an everlasting and most auspicious telekinetic effect. Therefore, many relevant stories about Lord Krsna have been provided and cross referenced within this manuscript; giving readers a priceless opportunity to begin engaging the mind in the highest yogic frequencies. It is a fact that who ever learns about the glories and pastimes of Lord Krsna is immediately freed from all material miseries! So seize this opportunity to begin washing all of your anxieties away, to purifying your heart, karma and your entire world with this metaphysical anecdote. It is the author's sincere hope that countless souls will be liberate, enlightened and saved from destruction by this transcendental information. In this age of *Kali-yuga,* the time of great misfortune and peril, it is more critical than ever for us all to begin purifying our karma and hearts for that journey back to the supreme spiritual abode. Nobody needs to be left behind in this *Rapture back to Godhead,* and miss out on the priceless opportunity to master the timeless sublime secrets of true psychokinesis.

This manuscript specifically shows you how to pragmatically enhance your own telekinetic powers for any purpose desired. In that sense, this is quite different from other works on the subject, which do not give the readers much inside information on how to control this powerful mental force and apply it to life itself! The amazing results of my private controlled PK experiments with the FP are published in chapter eleven. During this research, the stark reality of the FP and all mind over matter in general is unequivocally proven. My extensive empirical research records for the FP are also presented for you to study and contemplate in chapter nine. Analyzing the research and experimentation is crucial for taking your understanding of mind over matter and ultimate reality to the deepest level.

This manuscript is important in this *information age* because it presents cases of true PK. So many people all over the world are increasingly enamored with psi. Unfortunately, cases of true PK are so rare that they don't know how it really works at all. As a result, they also have no clue how to engage psi/PK forces to benefit their lives, but this manuscript solves that problem! The key to controlling your well of PK power is to understand how it functions by nature and its true divine or "cosmic"origins. I contend that the lack of knowledge about True PK is a void in life for which there is virtually no substitute. That is why manuscripts such as this are literally life savers for so many readers.

This manuscript should intrigue anybody interested in the supernatural, the field of psi (ESP, clairvoyance, premonition, telepathy and PK), parapsychology, occult science, action at a distance, yoga and metaphysics in general. Many people are scouring the globe tirelessly, spending ungodly sums of money, in search for that hard-core proof for the existence of mind over matter phenomenon, and in search of ultimate reality. Others are busy canvassing the planet with technologies of all sorts basically all only for the sake of studying the properties of subtle mental forces and their influences. Mind over matter through PK is optimized and even directly controlled when the right spiritual and psychological conditions are somehow created. Through my journeys, adventures in life, spiritual advancements and yogic conditioning, I inadvertently stumbled upon the mystery, treasure and the secrets for controlling PK. That is what gave birth to this manuscript.

God has empowered me to share these secrets and breakthroughs with the world. It is all for the sake of teaching others to help themselves and create whatever they want in their lives. The next logical step after recognizing that any source of power undeniably exists is learning how to work with it. The most crucial thing to know about PK is that it is certainly not any ordinary material energy. We are dealing with a very real force that specifically and directly control matter! The fact that this force in unquestionably real gives us confidence that it can in fact be put to work in our lives.

In the quest for solutions to life's most complex problems and knowledge of the highest grade, the secret information about PK is indispensable. It represents the next level of human evolution. There will always be the haves and the have nots, the sheep and the goats, the powerful and the powerless. In the final analysis, "only the fittest of the fittest shall survive," and yoga is centrally concerned with the concept of survival as a human being. Since our own intelligence is limited and is not adequate enough to handle all of our needs perfectly, it is most intelligent to use a higher power that is more intelligent as your agent.

This book discusses this intelligent force in depth, and it instructs readers on how to engage it in their lives for the highest blessings and benefits. In addition to presenting PK and concrete evidence for its existence, this book presents theories about how this force can be effectively used for self help, karmic repair, astral projection, personal achievement, spiritual realization and controlled transmigration into future lives (within the context of reincarnation). Additionally, this literature provides neophytes in the areas of transcendentalism, occult science, metaphysics and yoga with solid grounding and experiences in these areas. It gives readers the proof they have been seeking for so long about the reality of the supernatural. Finally there is bright light at the end of a very long tunnel of confusion and doubt regarding the mind's power.

There is a lot of misinformation in the world about how to become spiritually awakened and empowered. This book informs you about why it is vital to seek the aid of a spiritual master--a Guru who can give you access to God's secret treasures. Without the grace of my Gurus, I never could have made my most important advancements in life. In this book you can read about how my fortuitous encounters with my Gurus lead me to the ultimate reality.

Please note at the outset that there are those who are enlightened and fortunate enough to see the truth for what it really is. On the other hand, there are those that simply do not have the karmic capacity for doing so. Again, this work is only a result of my actual hands on experiences and personal involvements with "True-PK." I was drawn to the domain of PK not by my own choice but by divine providence.

This Is PK teaches readers how to think like professional PK practitioners for controlling life to the fullest. Only the most natural and real cases of PK are provided here along with some eye witness testimonies. False or "staged PK" will not do anything for helping you to understand how it works in reality. Thus, it is most important for you to learn about PK from a spiritual master, a yogi and saint who will not mislead. If you can not understand how PK and mind over matter works, then how can you learn to control it? Control over matter is one of the most desirable of all human attributes, and this next level of evolutionary thought is at your fingertips. This handbook book naturally fosters a heightened self-awareness and an elevated consciousness.

This kind of information is sometimes quite difficult to grasp for some only because it is often presented in obscure and incoherent ways. This handbook provides the information in a way that anybody can grasp and use with ease and efficiency. It gives you coveted and well guarded secrets that the highest mystics have used for controlling material nature to the fullest. Studying this manuscript is important for sense making in an "atomic age" that is increasingly influenced by metaphysics and psychology as scientific disciplines. The moment we conceded that the mind does function on a subatomic level which controls PK and physical matter, the field of psychology is pulled into the purview of mainstream science.

By properly integrating the mind control techniques provided here, anybody can learn to control matter and influence the revelry of reality with ease. Readers are given the tools for understanding our true spiritual nature, inner potential, and the realities of their own telekinetic powers. Aside from exposing the realities of true PK and clarifying common misconceptions, this book is intended to serve as a resource for self improvement, yogic advancement, and holistic health. By learning to control matter with the divine cosmic energy, people can easily witness all of their deepest dreams and desires unfolding right before their very eyes.

This manuscript certainly sheds light on many questions such as: Can human beings exploit certain mental forces that really effect material things? How can we begin to use more of the brain's potential, like Albert Einstein suggested? What is PK force, how can it be controlled and productively used to improve life and the world at large?

PK research covers more than a third of a century and involves people from diverse backgrounds and nations. The possibility of mind over matter has been demonstrated by many spontaneous paranormal occurrences reported over time. People traditionally have assumed a connection between the paranormal and mind over matter.

Since the spiritual revolution, many alternative opinions for PK were posited by material scientists This bunch of scientists claimed that PK has nothing to do with spiritual forces at all. This book attempts to shows readers that those views posited by material scientists are grossly inaccurate. They are based on a misunderstanding of ultimate reality, and deprivation of the absolute truth embedded within the world's most authoritative scriptures. Readers easily learn within this manuscript how to unleash the divine energy ("Shaktipat") within themselves. This fosters individualized experiences leading them to the ultimate reality, and the highest yogic initiations known as "Diksha." This critical spiritual initiation opens up a whole new world for all who are blessed to receive it. Your life will never be the same after reading this book because it automatically starts this initiation process by activating the Kundalini coiled up at the base of your spine. Many of you can already feel energetic changes happening as you continue reading. This approach to "awakening the snake"is easy and most highly recommended over other potentially unsafe methods. Meditating on this transcendental material definitely triggers important spiritual responses, as the chakras become gradually purified and tuned up!

The inherent and inseparable connections between science, technology, mysticism and spirituality are well established in the field of modern "psi research." One of the major hurdles for many in understanding the absolute truth is that science, the psychology of mysticism, and yoga have traditionally been studied separately in the

West. However, this has changed radically over the past century. By the turn of the twentieth century researchers were already using quite sophisticated apparatus for evaluating psychic and paranormal phenomenon. This handbook presents many of these research studies, and also analysis them within the context of spiritual science. As scientific technology advances as a whole, the methods, process and approaches for evaluating the supernatural progress commensurately. This manuscript exposes readers to various modern sophisticated technological approaches for studying PK. It provides a wealth of intriguing information on how PK has indeed been experimentally proven.

If you have any doubts about the realities and existence of PK, there are innumerable scientific articles, books, monographs and other research studies for you to find the truth presented once again. Before making any critical decision, you must have sufficient facts, and this book is here to guide you in the right direction. Since mind over matter is clearly the most important skill in life, this is the most critical decision that you will ever make in your entire life--to believe or not to believe in the power of your mind's PK force.

Implications of recent PK discoveries are quite far-reaching, to say the least, because they have unlimited potential. In fact, many international researchers and scientists consider these psi discoveries more important than that of nuclear energy. By integrating my personal hands on experience and knowledge in PK with the formal analysis of academic researchers, we are able to understand how it works in a whole new light. In any new area of scientific discovery, formal academic research is conducted, which is then integrated with the experiences of everyday people.

In Principle, nothing is discovered without someone observing it during related work, and it being further confirmed experimentally. For example, Einstein discovered nuclear energy while engaged in that area of study and analysis. Thomas Edison discovered the functioning principle (FP) for the lightbulb only while engaged in studying electricity. Christopher Columbus supposedly discovered the New World. In any case, his "Eureka" only happened while he was engaged in sailing across the oceans. Likewise, I discovered the FP only while engaged in the acquisition of the highest transcendental yogic and occult knowledge.

Many exciting breakthroughs in the field of PK have occurred during various types of religious and spiritual practices, such as the seance settings in the Victorian era. My personal experience has proven to me that the highest understanding comes about through the practice of the mystical royal yoga. This book explains to you all about how to work on that most sublime metaphysical pathway. Its most potent spiritual energies give rise to PK phenomenon of the highest grade. Most modern researchers are totally baffled about how this force can be used on a practical level. The author believes that the most powerful application of PK energy is using its manifestations as an opportunity to disseminate the Absolute Truth about Lord Sri Krsna (Pronounced "Krishna"). As far as I am concerned, the so-called skeptics of PK are plainly foolish and rather ignorant because all of my experiences, research findings, discoveries and breakthroughs are quite consistent with modern psi researchers. They are not in accordance with anything that the so-called skeptics have to say about the nature of PK.

This book shows you how to use yogic precept for understanding PK Force to the fullest, and controlling it for any purpose desired. Many readers are in positions of pressing need or great trouble that calls for immediately effective solutions, and this information is ideal for those purposes. If your back is up against the wall, and it seems like there is no hope in the world. Or, if you are in trouble and need quick and highly effective solutions, then this book will certainly bring you immediate help directly from the spiritual world! Remember that delay is the enemy, so don't wait for the right time to start using your new secret karmic power!

Whether or not you happen to share my exact same spiritual views is not relevant in your ability to learn a new yogic survival skill. Everybody should learn about recent discoveries concerning this distinct semi-physical force (PK) that the mind can apparently control for any purpose. God has given man free will, so I can only provide suggestions about how this sub-atomic force should be used. I can only try to show you in this manuscript that PK is unequivocally real, that this has been proven scientifically; and all of this is supported by the greatest spiritual masters that have ever lived. In addition my own personal research published in this book with corroborate the existence of a creature known as PK.

The rest is your free will. You can have anything that you want by understanding the functioning principles for controlling this energy both consciously and unconsciously. Many layman from all walks of life, on both spiritual and religious paths, have learned the most powerful keys and the secrets to life itself from Gurus like myself, from saints, sages, rishis and other "spiritual adepts." This secret knowledge is the highest and most effective source of self help, improvement and spiritual liberation. As you will observe throughout this book, the greatest PK agents of all times have been trained within the sacred context of the "Guru-Disciple relationship."

I am no exception to that rule, so you also will read about my experiences with real Gurus. Recall that a Guru is only a teacher and a disciple a student; and that this relationship is specially arranged by God, "The Father" of everything. It is protected, blessed and empowered by His hand. Everybody is welcome here for learning how to develop and use telekinetic power. Even atheistic people can also learn about how to take better control over the divine cosmic forces and attain what they consider the "impersonal" supreme reality. The Siddhartha Gautama (Buddha) is classic historical proof that even the greatest atheists can indeed create healthy spiritual lives and higher powers. In other words, we simply should not allow for sectarian thinking to cloud our rationality, and destroy the opportunity of a lifetime–the chance to master the secrets of true psychokinesis!

Chapter 1. Briefing on Psychokinesis

The study of psychic phenomenon (psi) concerns events that are inexplicable under present knowledge of psychology or physics. Psi phenomenon involves the interactions between organisms and their environment that are not controlled by any known sensory-motor systems. The primary areas of psi are survival research, ESP, clairvoyance, precognition, and psychokinesis. Survival research involves the search for proof of some form of survival after physical death. For example, near death experiences are studied in this field. ESP is the process of acquiring information and knowledge without using any of the five senses. Researchers have consistently concluded that ESP involves elements of PK and vice versa. Telepathy is the ability to know thoughts within the mind of another person. Clairvoyance is awareness of a scene or object even when it is not known to another person, and telepathy is ruled out. Precognition enables one to peer into the future, and considerable Experimental evidence indicates that this possibly does occur in humans. This book specifically concerns the study of psychokinesis, which is the ability to transfer energy into another person, or an object such as a refrigerator.

Mind over matter manifests in unlimited ways that can be studied and observed within the context of psi research. Psychokinesis was referred to as "telekinesis" prior to J.B. Rhine's impact and discoveries within the field. In addition, telekinesis pertains more to subtle energetic small scale changes in material particles under the mind's control, instead of more apparent and observable effects. By contrast, PK refers to more large scale and observable changes in physical matter such as spoon-bending or the lifting of automobiles in times of danger. PK is the propensity of matter to be influenced by the mind, whether intentionally or inadvertently. Because of its unlimited potential, PK is now the most actively researched area in the realm of parapsychology. It is nothing less than mind over matter and concerns the ability to move or affect a physical situation or object without the use of any physical contact or intermediary. For example, something happens to an object in your environment, and you do not physically make it happen. No muscular effort is involved, and yet a person makes it happen in some other paranormal, mental and nonphysical way.

PK concerns the paranormal ability to effect the activity of matter by mental intention (or perhaps another aspect of mental activity) alone. It is a specific form of mind over matter that is often   produced by remote invisible means. In fact, since 2004 the term "remote influencing" is being commonly used to characterize certain kinds of psychokinesis. Accounts of PK have been recorded since the remotest of times. These cases involve levitation, spontaneous healing, and supernatural phenomena attributed to "holy ones" and spiritual adepts all over the world. Many people believe that PK force is the distinct energy that every magician, healer, and occultist relies on to manifest physical results.

PK also involves moving objects from one place to another with no physical contact. It also means deformation of objects by using mental energies, such as bending a spoon or a key. The term "psychokinesis" was derived from the Greek terms "psyche" meaning life or soul and "kinesis" which means to move. It literally means "distant movement" and is the more frequently used term today for what was formerly called telekinesis. Scientists from various backgrounds and disciplines maintain that there is sufficient evidence of psychokinesis in controlled experiments to corroborate its existence, which justifies it as a field of study.

True PK is related to the mystical powers of shamans, yogis, magicians, witches, saints, poltergeist and especially "acts of God." One hundred years ago, investigators of such claims began to devise special scientific methods of studying them. Over time this highly specialized information resonated in the field of psi and psychical research. Due to its highly specialized nature, most findings and discoveries in PK research have been easily overlooked by the general public. However, this massive ignorance has no bearing on the bottom line, which is the reality of mind over matter. It is only through mediums such as this manuscript that the keys to life are provided, by exposing the truth about this divine force that anybody can learn how to control.   Physical energy is created by electromagnetic impulses. Universal life force energy, or psychic energy, is called "prana." In psychokinesis, one taps into prana energy and then combines it with physical energy.

A large body of literature is now devoted to the study of PK, particularly within the scientific and psychology communities. There are even technologies called psychotronics available that most people find quite effective for amplifying and controlling their psychokinetic powers (for example visit, and check out these exciting products). Apparently, this force can be either controlled consciously or unconsciously, with results that may or may not be obvious to observers. PK is generally viewed as the proclivity of the mind to manipulate matter, time, space, or energy through means quite impossible by currently understood laws of physics.

The myriad forms and manifestations of PK may also include: The movements of static objects across counters and tabletops; the tipping of tables and levitating of other large furniture during seances; causing mental visualizations to appear on photographic film; producing glowing lights in rooms out of nowhere; swinging pendulums in sealed containers; creating drastic temperature fluctuations in rooms; affecting lights and other electronics such as refrigerators and automobiles; bilocation; levitation; and spontaneous healing. Electrokinesis is the psi ability to control electrons at any distance which often results in one being able to mentally control electrical apparatus such as car lights, light bulbs, refrigerators, and computers. This very rare ability is also manifested in the ability to produce lightening and extremely powerful thunderstorms by influencing electric particles.

A classic example of PK has been reported by many people throughout history, where a clock stops at the exact moment of one's death. PK can manifest powerful physical changes in subatomic particles, chemical compositions, electromagnetic and temperature changes, alterations in plant growth, changes in the behaviors and bodily processes of certain animals (i.e. fish and mice) changes in physical objects, and perhaps body changes including miraculous healing. Of psychic abilities, "true PK" is indeed one of the most rare.

As a general rule, very few people have been able to demonstrate this ability in the presence of others, nor have they had any real first-hand experiences with it. This book was only written book because I am definitely an exception to that general rule. Therefore, I am coming from a totally different perspective in life that I believe has the power to change lives. Psychokinesis can be used to distort or move an object, or to influence certain devices designed to detect it such as a "telekinetic wheel." The fascinating thing about the FP presented in chapter eight is how it directly manifests through a modern technology in ways that enables us to monitor, understand, and perhaps control PK energy in a whole new way.

In the field of PK, there are two basic types of measurable and observable effects. Micro-PK more closely is associated with telekinesis, while macro PK is connected to psychokinesis. However, the terms are often used synonymously and interchangeably. In micro-PK, the effects are subtle, and very small such as the manipulation of molecules, atoms, electrons, subatomic particles, etc. This can be measured using certain scientific apparatus such as random number generators, magnometers, or dice roll machines.

Micro-PK may also include the power to influence temperature, magnetic fields affecting the chemical constitution of a photograph, which is known as "psychic photography" or "thoughtaugraphy." As an example, Ted Serios was researched heavily for his telekinetic ability to willfully create PK influences on film, especially while he was intoxicated. On the other hand, Macro-PK is a large-scale effect that can be easily observed. Examples of this include lifting of large objects such as automobiles, bending of metals, breaking petrified coconuts by merely using the palm of ones hand (Iron Palm), levitation, and teleportation of objects.

Over the past century, parapsychologists have made astounding discoveries about the human mind and its capabilities. There now exists ample evidence indicating that by mere conscious desire (wishing), unconscious intent, and by will power, humans can indeed influence physical matter in their environment and at great distances. At this point, modern researchers especially in the West universally concur that they do not know how this is possible. Modern scientists are unclear about what laws govern its operation, and why humans were endowed with such an ability in the first instance. Based on my work in this area, I know for certain that there is some subtle force that can control matter, which specifically reacts to our thoughts and emotions. This handbook sheds light on these issues, while it analyze PK through a lense that is quite different from mainstream-orthodox Western science. I believe that this will give readers a deeper understanding of what we are actually dealing with.

In remote times, the great sages, rishis, philosophers and Brahmanas would hold endless discourse about the relationships between the mind, body, and the "external" world. For centuries, scientists, philosophers and other scholars have been keenly aware of the possibility of mind over matter. By the middle ages, scientists knew that some force hidden within man's mind could be summoned, triggered, activated and directed by will power. In fact, Francis Bacon published a work entitled *Sylva Sylarum* in 1561, where he wrote that there is some kind of physical force within man's mind that could be tested upon things that have the "lightest and the easiest motion, such as the coming up of herbs or upon their bending one way or another, or upon the casting of dice."

In another one of Bacon's works entitled The New Atlantis, he said that the "motions of shuffling cards or casting of dice" can be used to "test the binding of thoughts." The use of probability theory to study deviations from statistically and theoretically expected chance outcomes was introduced by Charles Richet, a French Nobel Laureate. Incidentally, he was heavily involved with PK research and worked closely studying the notorious Italian PK practitioner Eusapia Pallidino.

The 14th century PK analysis from Frances Bacon mentioned above are quite prophetic for a few reasons. Only a few centuries later in the 1930's and 1940's, PK was studied scientifically in dice-throwing experiments conducted by J.B. Rhine at Duke University. Rhine successfully proved in these experiments that subjects could mentally influence the landing of dice throws causing them to land with a particular number more often than chance accounts for. Rhine also proved that the mind can really exert a physical force and project it into the environment even at a distance. This is discussed much more extensively in chapter five. Another ironic aspect of Bacon's theory is that Dr. Bernard Grad, a biochemist from McGill University in Montreal, Canada has recently proven irrefutably that mental will power can affect plant and herb growth, which is discussed further in chapter seven.

Many people hesitate to accept mind over matter mainly because they believe it is childish or silly. As children growing up, our imaginations were wild, and "magic" was something that we had first hand experience with. This was this frame of mind that formed the very basis of our whole lives. We knew that it was real, and as we assimilated into the so-called real world, we lost track of this frame of mind and its inherent power. Mind over matter is now a scientifically provable hypothesis. It is a well established scientific fact that the more intelligent humans are constantly working with.
The vast majority of people never even contemplate PK or its implications. However, a rare few can not avoid its manifestations in their every day lives and our karma forces us to deal with it.

Many people are increasingly growing interested in the connections between the sub-atomic world of physics and the phenomenal world of collective sensory experience. To most people the concept of mind over matter is familiar, but merely an idea with no basis in reality, similar to science fiction. However, if it was conclusively and scientifically determined that humans could influence matter using the mind alone, the tone of our whole age would drastically change and take on whole new dimensions.

Although these issues have been addressed in modern times by relatively few people, they have been extensively tested under careful and professional experimental conditions. This testing has generated evidence which appears to suggest that the mind has a distinct force that responds to thought, and directly influences the disposition of physical matter. This seems to be a natural mental ability, yet a very hidden and underdeveloped one in nearly everybody, except for a few "enlightened" or especially gifted ones among us.

All of this experimental evidence has resonated in the field of parapsychology under the classification of PK. It has exploded into the fastest growing area of research in the field of parapsychology primarily because it presents such new horizons for science. Anything that presents the possibility for unprecedented change naturally evolves into an area of major research, discovery, and development. Even in light of all overwhelming evidence proving the existence of PK, and despite some personal experiences with it, people still hesitate to accept it. This apprehension is mainly based on fear of total and complete change, which often threatens our psychological comfort zones. Embracing mind over matter with its far reaching implications creates some level of confusion about how it works. The central purpose of this handbook and its yogic knowledge is to provide you with transcendental insight about how PK works, what it really means, and what this cosmic force is doing right now on our planet!

Chapter 2: Real Yoga and True-PK

This chapter educates readers on the nature and purpose of real yoga. This is vital to understand because my most profound discoveries in PK and mind over matter only happened as a result of engaging in disciplinary yoga. So it is important for people to know something about the true meaning and structure of yoga, especially while trying to develop and enhance their own mind over matter abilities. This chapter helps you to understand how practicing transcendental yoga can lead to you perfection, mastery over life itself, and powerful control over material nature.

It is clear that interest in yoga is increasing at an unprecedented rate all around the world. Some of us have noticed yoga studios, organizations and similar "societies" sprouting up from every direction. People are fairly confused about this sudden international phenomenon, and I hope to shed some light on the subject. The first thing to recognize is that your concept of yoga itself very well could be erroneous. That requires you to literally dump all preconceived notions regarding yoga from your mind, and then learn about the absolute truth on the subject.

This yoga trend, so to speak, is largely a result of the information age and its impact on international trade, communication and interchange. Along the way, truth, and vital information from the source gets passed along, tainted, and naturally corrupted. This information is then passed down into societies that honestly can not distinguish between what is artificial and what is real. Just like religious principles that have been disseminated throughout the world from one source (the Vedas) and fragmented into different so-called truths, yoga has experienced structural and doctrinal breakdown over time and geography. This naturally fosters misunderstanding about what it really means

Yoga literally means "union," and its techniques were originally developed in India to enable the practitioner to attain union with the supreme reality (God). Its fundamental purpose is for the yogi to attain independence from the external influences of both nature and man! That is indeed a very lofty objective. It is also designed to help us achieve a state of detachment from internal emotions, tensions, and other obstacles to the ideal states of self-sufficiency. That is why yoga is the best approach for those of us who are interested in self-help. The doctrines and scriptures of yoga are so pervasive that they permeate all religious schools in India, and the entire region of countries surrounding it including China, Tibet, and Nepal.

Doctrines such as yoga that are extremely widespread naturally develop into various sects, belief systems, denominations and schools of thought. This explains why traces of valuable yogic philosophies are found in schools of Buddhism such as reincarnation. If we use a spectrum to illustrate the various forms of yoga, on one end of the scale would be that form which is solely concerned with physical well-being and physical health such as Hatha Yoga. The intermediate part of the spectrum would represent the yoga principally concerned with emotional and mental health such as *Laya-yoga*. On the other far end of the continuum, the object is spiritual perfection and personal autonomy, which is reflected in the science of Bhakti Yoga.

The final stages of yoga are characterized by the insatiable desire for union with God. All other yogic practices are really supposed to be stepping stones leading to that point where one wills to associate with Lord Sri Krsna, who is known as the "Supreme Personality of Godhead." Traditionally, yoga involves breathing exercises, mystical incantations known as mantras, and specific behavioral injunctions for disciplinary purposes and mind control. In principle, yoga is concerned with our survival, spiritual elevation in this human life, and ultimately the cessation of material existence.

Yoga was developed 8,000 years ago as a pure spiritual science for devotion to God. In the West, it tends to be associated with physical health and psychological influence rather than for spiritual elevation. This is gradually changing because of the information age creating greater awareness in the West about the higher forms of yoga and their underlying purposes. Since everything in our lives and existence is really mental/spiritual, it is crucial to use yoga for what it is intended--spiritual empowerment.

One of the best kept occult secrets is that practicing the higher forms of yoga is the most effective way for conditioning the mind to effectively control and influence matter. My own breakthroughs in the field of PK never started, until after I renewed my divine consciousness through practicing transcendental yoga. So, when you are seeking the ultimate verities within the field of metaphysics or the occult science, you need not look outside of authoritative yogic scriptural information for the "Absolute Truth." In fact, the core pillars for metaphysics and the occult science are based on yogic precepts. That is why many phenomenal telekinetic discoveries and effects are constantly experienced by transcendentalists and yogis of all varieties.

Interestingly enough, expansion in the field of PK and mind over matter in general seems to be increasing proportionally with that of yoga around the world. For example, we see interest in yoga at an all time high in the very same way that interest in PK has made it the most hotly researched area in the field of parapsychology. The essence of mind over matter is true yoga, as it pertains to the fabric of reality itself. There are various forms of yoga designed to influence different aspects of reality as we know it. Yogic practices and processes are primarily based on the principles within the Patanjali system. Through the process of disciplinary yoga, one gradually becomes detached from the material concept of life. This fosters a state of trance known as *Samadhi*.

When referring to yoga, we really mean the process of linking our minds and souls with the Supreme Absolute Truth. The ultimate perfection of all yoga naturally should be our aim. According to the Vedas, the most authoritative world scriptures on yoga and real religion, this transcendental plane of perfection is known as *Bhakti-yoga* or "Krsna Consciousness." According to His Divine Grace A.C. Bhaktivedanta Swami Prabhupada (Srila Prabhupada), the Founder of International Society for Krishna Consciousness (ISKCON), nothing in existence can excel Bhakti Yoga because it is full of spiritual knowledge. Since spiritual energy is of the highest and most potent grade, nothing can surpass this form of yoga. Bhakti literally means direct service unto Lord Sri Krsna. Its main purpose is to bring Him enjoyment and ecstatic pleasure. It is the perfection of life itself and all yoga, which should naturally be everybody's aim. When one has attained the perfection of yoga, one is always engaged in Samadhi. This is a fact which is confirmed by Lord Sri Krsna in the *Bhagavad-Gita.*

Samadhi is a transcendental level of consciousness, where we can experiences the supreme reality and become self-realized souls. This state occurs when the topmost chakra (Sahasrara) is activated. It is a fact that most people including yogis never achieve Samadhi during this entire life. Many lives, many masters and incarnations are required before the energy elevates to this apex. However, with good enough fortune, and through the practice of Bhakti, one can easily attain this sublime state in this lifetime. Samadhi is complete absorption is God-Consciousness. Recall that before you can become "absorbed in God Consciousness," you must have the insatiable desire to unite with Him via yoga. By definition samadhi means of "fixed mind." According to the Nirukti, the Vedic dictionary, "when the mind is fixed for understanding the self, it is said to be in Samadhi." That is not possible for those who are too obsessed with sense gratification and deluded by that materialism.

According to the *Bhagavad-gita*, Chapter 6, Texts 20-23:

"In the stage of perfection called trance, or samadhi, one's mind is completely restrained from material mental activities by practice of yoga. This perfection is characterized by one's ability to see the self by the pure mind and to relish and rejoice in the self. In that joyous state, one is situated in boundless transcendental happiness, realized by through transcendental senses." Established thus, one never departs from the truth, and upon gaining this he thinks there is no greater gain. Being situated in such a position, one is never shaken, even in the midst of greatest difficulty. This indeed is actual freedom from all miseries arising from material contact."

Samadhi is marked by an increase and intensification in PK phenomenon of all sorts in your life and environment. There are varying degrees of samadhi, depending on the degree of activation and the type of yoga one is engaged in. In the Patanjali system, there are two distinct stages of samadhi. One is known as *samrajnata-samadhi*, and the other stage is *asamprajnata-samadhi.* The former stage is attained through various philosophical processes that situate one on a transcendental plane of consciousness.

When the later level is achieved, there are no longer any entanglements with mundane pleasure, as the mind is transcendental to all gratification arising from the senses. When one achieves this transcendental level, one can not be moved from it. Yogis that are unable to reach this state of advancement are considered unsuccessful. One advantage to practicing *bhakti-yoga* is that even if a bhakta is unsuccessful, he will be elevated to a higher planet in the next life. Lord Sri Krsna confirms this in the *Bhagavad-gita* and never waivers from any promise He makes the His devotees. You would be surprised how many people I have spoken to who have the *Bhagavad-Gita* sitting at home on the book shelf, and they have no idea what it purports. Well, I think its time to familiarize yourself with this ageless yogic wisdom that comes directly from the mouth of God.

Samadhi is indeed a sign of attaining this victory over matter. We should remember that it is the very essence of yoga, not merely the highest yogic technique. Vyasa the incarnation of the Lord who was empowered to disseminate the Vedas regarded yoga and Samadhi as synonymous. That is evident by his statement: "Yogah Samadhi." My discovery of the FP occurred around the same time that I began entering into this sublime state through yoga.

The state of samadhi is one of the end goals of all yogic pursuits. When this perfection of yoga is attained, one is always absorbed in trance. In contrast with two distinct forms of samadhi in the Patanjali system, there is another way of conceptualizing of it that consists of three distinct stages: 1) True concentration, 2) Meditation, and 3) Samadhi. In the first phase of true concentration, there are no longer find any physiological, chemical, or physical basis for the yogi's "operations." In the Western world, this is studied within the field of psi. The yogi's operations involve "unconditioned mental dynamics" that are generally unknown to the world of Western science and psychology.

Upon realizing that there is some definite source of supreme power creating great miracles that the yogi can not control, he naturally moves on to next the state of "mediation." This state is connected with the initial form of samadhi in the Pantanjali system, as it leads to immense philosophical insight and introspection connected with the yogi's new awakening. Another natural reaction of this stage is that the yogi learns to control this power! In meditation state, the goal is to gradually wield control over the physical plane. That is achieved by learning to control "Psi Plasma," which is just another term for the prana life energy used by some researchers including the prominent neuro-physiologist Dr. Andrija Puharich. Prana is directly and unquestionably associated with the "divine serpent power" known as Kundalini.

This divine energy gives rise to PK phenomenon of all sorts. There are various ways of manifesting this form of control, and levitation is one example. When I reached the state of meditation on the Supreme Lord Sri Krsna, the FP happened with much more intensity because I learned to control it. In the first stage, I merely noticed many paranormal things happening including the FP. This shows that I attained increased control over the divine Kundalini through TM. It is likely that what we regard as mind over matter effects in the West are perhaps only a label for manifestations of awakened Kundalini.

After acquiring these supernatural and paranormal powers, the yogi becomes conditioned to enter samadhi. There is no comparable term in the Western world to help us apprehend what it really means. That is why first hand personalized experience is indispensable for understanding these spiritual processes. This book should help readers to have their own experiences in this area, and hence discover the truth for themselves. The final stage of samadhi is characterized by the yogi realizing himself as a nuclear mental entity that can control the physical dimensions of his body, affect physical objects at a distance from his body, and is able to move freely as a mobile center of consciousness independently of his body. That is the real meaning of the independence and autonomy achieved through the practice of mystical yoga. This high level of "independence" manifests in the form of astral adventures and journeys into many other worlds.

The phase of samadhi coronates with the final stage in the Patanjali system, which represents union with God. My hope that all of my disciples and readers experience samadhi in its richest form. Those that are distracted by the by-products of yoga such as miracles are unable to proceed and advance to the state of "perfection" referred to above in Chapter 6 Texts 20-23 cited above from the *Bhagavad-Gita*. Miracles are only the conscious stimulation of more patterns of reality than are generally observable under the linear-analytic Newtonian lens. Along these lines, William Blake advises:

"May God us keep
From single vision
and Newton's sleep."

Those engaged in the practice of supernatural feats for entertainment or other mundane purposes should note that the objective of yoga (attaining perfection) is completely lost in this manner. That is why my PK discoveries are not used to entertain or appease others. According to the Vedas, the best method for attaining the highest state of perfection in life is through *bhakti -yoga*. In terms of making the highest spiritual and religious connection that is even more powerful then miracles, the *Bhagavad-Gita* provides in Chapter 8, Text 12:

" The yogic situation is that of detachment from all sensual engagements. Closing the doors of the senses and fixing the mind on the heart and the life air at the top of the head, one establishes himself in yoga. "

The next scripture states that whoever at the time of death focuses his prana energy (life air)on the third eye (*ajna chakra*) and uses the strength of yoga to remember Lord Sri Krsna will certainly make it back His Supreme Abode. This verse is exceptionally important for understanding the highest application of our PK powers. Even if we acquire all of the material things that we desire on Earth or any other planet in the material world, we can not stay here forever. Hence, we must learn from the Lord about how to situate our consciousness on a transcendental level, when we leave these physical bodies. The system of *sat-cakra-yoga* is particularly useful in this respect. Here Lord Krsna advises Arjuna to fix the "life air" (Prana) between the eyes and remember Him in the Shyamasundara form, which is God's original form.

This is yet another superb description of how *sat-cakra-yoga* works to control our consciousness in this life and prepare it for the next. The ajna chakra, is known as the "control center" as it relates specifically to developing a strong and independent mind. Ajna literally means command, as this chakra can only be awakened via command or will power. It is also known as the seat of the "inner Guru," who must command or will for the Kundalini to move past this energy vortex. In other words, we must act as our own internal Guru, and do what Krsna says by using the "strength of yoga," and will power to make the life air move through this center, particularly at the moment of death.

This third eye vortex is also associated with the feminine aspect of the divine. This "divine feminine energy" is known as Shakti in the schools of mystical yoga, which symbolizes the consort of Lord Vishnu. That is another example of how the timeless knowledge from the Vedas has passed down into other religious believe systems. This energy represents ideal union with God in yoga. This explains why Lord Sri Krsna admonishes Arjuna to focus on the ajna chakra at the moment of death. Unfortunately most people in the world have falsely associated God only with the quality of manhood or masculinity. This has understandably created lots of feminist ideals including goddess worship. Now you can see that the feminine aspect of the Supreme Lord and Controller is inherent and indispensable.

It is very prudent to develop a strong connection with this divine telekinetic force through transcendental yoga. Of course, many other spiritual activities also activate the ajna chakra including meditation, prayer, chanting, contemplation, and visualization. The active quality of Shakti explains why the ajna chakra center is directly connected with developing mystical powers and paranormal abilities. Another notable aspect of these verses is how Lord Sri Krsna instructs His disciple Arjuna to focus on Him by the "strength of yoga," with an "undeviating mind." What does Krsna mean by "the 'strength' of yoga?"

Here, Lord Sri Krsna explains to His disciple Arjuna on the battlefield how the system of sat-cakra-yoga works in practice. Many people including one of my very own Gurus concede that they have no idea how chakra yoga works. Practicing *bhakti-yoga* causes the prana to focus on the heart chakra, which causes this life energy to naturally drift up to the topmost chakras. That is a key concept for attaining enlightenment. This is a different approach to raising the kundalini energy than most people are used to. Most people are accustomed to the idea of the kundalini being coiled up at the base of the spine, and gradually moving upwards through all of the chakras as it purifies them. Again, the problem with this approach is that most people are unable to get their kundalini to reach the upmost chakras in this life time. And, that accounts for all of the yogis who have not seen the supreme.

Since we are discussing PK, it can not be overlooked how Lord Sri Krsna performed the most impressive mind over matter feats. A classic example is where he demonstrated superior psychokinetic strength by lifting *Govardhan Hill* with only one hand as a little child! That is definitely analogous to what we consider a PK feat today in modern society such as lifting an automobile with one hand so save a person underneath; and that has happened on record! This lifting of the hill was done to save a large number of animals whose lives were threatened by a major flood. This perfectly illustrates the "strength of yoga" that He refers to in the *Bhagavad-gita*. As the creator everything, Lord Sri Krsna demonstrated the most extreme examples of yogic strength and power. By lifting Govardhana Hill with only one hand, the King of yoga Himself showed us that the strength of yoga is mind over matter, and psychokinetic power as well.

Again, many of us have heard about or witnessed instances where senior citizens have been able to lift automobiles including buses to save their loved ones trapped underneath. We accept these effects as being "psychokinetic" by nature, but they pale in comparison to the strength and power of yoga exhibited by Sri Krsna, when he lifted *Govardhana Hill*. That highlights the difference between the individual souls and the supreme soul! That is the difference between God and man.

Till this day, Govardhana Hill still stands to symbolize the sheer "strength" of yoga. I consider it the ultimate example of true-PK. I believe that the strength of yoga which Krsna refers to in the Gita is actually PK power, and that is why studying this handbook is so priceless. Whenever we speak of the most adept yogis, we refer to those like Satya Sai Baba or the Great Yogi Malarepa, who have exhibited strong telekinetic powers such as materialization phenomenon, yogic flying, bi-location, and levitation. As I espouse throughout the treatise, the highest application of yogic strength (PK) is to teleport our souls back to God's Kingdom.

Chanting the Holy Names of God, through the *Maha Mantra* is the easiest, most effective and sublime way of instantly harnessing the life energy within these higher chakras, and particularly within the heart realm: So chant *Hare Krsna Hare Krsna, Krsna Krsna Hare Hare Hare Rama Hare Rama Rama Rama Hare Hare!* Deep healing can happen within the realm of the heart chakra when we supply it with sufficient prana-- the vital life force. When we transcend the lower chakras through transcendental yoga , and arise to the vortex of the heart, there is only oneness with the divine, as our consciousness becomes dovetailed with God.

All theistic traditions believe that God is great. Lord Sri Krsna establishes His greatness consistently throughout Vedic literatures including the *Bhagavad-Gita*. He gave a glimpse of His infinite greatness by revealing his vishva-rupa darshana to Arjuna. That was one of the greatest mystical visions recorded in all world literature. I also consider it to be an extreme case of telekinesis where Arjuna saw within the Universal Form and everything in existence within Lord Krsna. He saw all the planets, the stars and universes and all living beings: celestial, terrestrial and subterranean. Krsna demonstrates his omnipotence by effortlessly vanquishing numerous demons such as Aghasura when He was only six years old. Krsna also destroyed Kesi and Kaliya, who all scourged of the universe.

True PK involves real paranormal phenomenon of the highest grade, rather than anything staged, televised or setup involving the sleight of hand. It is directly associated with superior spiritual powers. Until I discovered the FP through practicing disciplinary yoga, I had no idea that PK was real, and that the mind unquestionably has these supernatural abilities. I was one of the biggest skeptics that you could find. Naturally Lord Sri Krsna on Earth was in a position to exhibit the most powerful form of PK as God manifested in the flesh. He is also able to trigger PK in us more powerfully than anything else can. Anybody can develop these powers, but not to the extent of Krsna or His incarnations ("avatars"). The incarnations are not by any means ordinary human beings. We are directly appointed by the Lord to perform specific functions. The incarnations of the Lord are innumerable over time and space, and we all have different superhuman powers.

As the life energy rises to the higher chakras through worship of the Supreme Lord residing in the heart, it becomes very effective to work within the throat chakra for willing PK to function in specific ways. The reason why the throat chakra is considered the realm of powerful creation is because it controls PK by the element of will power. Creation is apparently quite feasible on the frequency of the throat chakra, while transmigration after life and astral projection are most easily achieved through the transcendental wavelengths of the brow chakra. The most important thing is to learn as much as you can about the chakras, how to tune into them, and what they represent. Then you can use your PK to greatly enhance all of these subjects realms of your life, and project that into the objective world.

Although the aim of human life is to transcend the lower chakras, it is critical not to neglect these vital centers. The concept of "living through the chakras" and within these realms is indeed quite powerful. We all are actually living out our karmas through the various chakra frequencies. Therefore, it is critical to understand and learn about what the chakras represent and begin applying your PK and will power towards specific chakras. By applying PK to any of the chakras, we galvanize them with the energy that is necessary for us to experience the best that chakra frequency has to offer. One of the main reasons for lots of suffering even among spiritual and religious people is only neglect of the chakras, which controls our karma.

Lord Sri Krsna Himself indirectly endorses living through the chakras, even up until the last moment of our lives. Throughout this book, you will observe how PK force has been measured, observed, and closely analyzed. You will see for yourself how it has been unequivocally proven to exist in various ways including the FP. Since we know that the mind can control this subtle force with ease, the best way to take life itself to a much higher dimension is to apply PK force directly into our chakras! This is indeed one of the highest forms of "self-help."

There are many ways of enhancing telekinetic abilities and understanding it better. Using chakra yoga as a mapping system for life is one of the best approaches. It is so valuable because the chakra system is one of the most ancient conceptual systems about our true nature. Combining that sacred Vedic knowledge with new discoveries about PK force can certainly have a dramatic effect on life. All of us have experienced damage to our chakras to some degree, which drastically affects our quality of life, health, well-being, emotional stability and mental clarity. I have found that chakra healing is one of the most beneficial applications of your PK.

Each chakra realm has a distinct purpose that endows us with different abilities. The brow chakra that Lord Sri Krsna is referring to is also related to the concept of "projection," and "astral projection," which is why He instructs using it to project the soul back to Him. By following this instruction from Krsna, you can easily achieve a spiritual existence in the anti-material world. Similarly, you can transfer yourself to any planet that you desire, by following certain yogic processes for doing so. For example, if you wish to go to the sun, the moon or any other planet, it is quite possible by following prescribed yogic methods. The best way to understand the power of chakra yoga is through hands-on experience, where you charge one of your chakras with prana energy, trigger specific changes, and then evaluate the results. Basically, you run a very safe test and experiment with your chakras. You will observe in this book how there is a world of difference between the experimental groups that are treated with PK and control groups in research that are not. Similarly, there is a world of difference between chakras that have been treated with PK and ones that have not. Just like a plant's whole life can be affected by this application of mind power, PK applied to your chakras can unquestionably change your whole life! First you must know more about PK and how to use it, which is the purpose of this manuscript.

The main thing to remember is that your chakras certainly represent your own distinct and subjective worlds. This is encompassed by certain concepts outlined in Mahayana Buddhist ideology. Buddhism went through major changes in India, after the philosopher Nagarjuna began propagating the Madhyamika doctrine (" the middle way") around the second century A.D. During this time, he was standing against the widespread Abhidharma belief, which states that the objective world and all its constituents including the individual should be considered as real entities. Nagarjuna posited a brilliant idea that the main error for humanity is positing the existence of an external objective world that is separate from his own subjective world.

Nagarjuna contended that there is nothing other than the "self," and the delusion that there is anything other than self is an error--a devil trap of Maya that most have fallen prey to. Nagarjuna termed this doctrine Prapanca (false imagination) and maintained that it is the source of all misery and suffering that mankind faces. In other words, man can not understand the world, as he draws artificial lines of demarcation and creates dichotomies between himself and the rest of the world through his actions, thoughts, and language.

This is historically what gave rise to the basic pillars of Madhyamika ideology, including the doctrine of Pratitya Sumatapada. This doctrine teaches that everything in the universe is interdependent and interrelated. Nagarjuna believed that by transcending our conditioned way of categorical reasoning, we reach the state of Nirvana, or liberation from worldly desires. This is what is meant by "the Void" in Buddhist thought this is typically misinterpreted in the Western world. The void does not mean "oblivion" or "nothingness," as most people believe, but rather the merging of our subjective differences with the whole which is absolute. It is most closely connected with the final state of Samadhi, where the thoughts are totally stilled.

Many people commonly misinterpret another Buddhistic notion, which states that if the mind and matter are one and the same. Most people think this doctrine purports that the mind should be able to totally control matter. First off, that is not possible because there is only one "Supreme Controller" who is God. So, what this doctrine really means is that there is a subjective part of our mental and spiritual being (i.e. the chakras, and our individual karma) that are non-different from the objective material world. Dr. J.B. Rhine supports this position in his views about PK, where he theorizes that man is composed of a nonphysical mental body that somehow controls the physical world.

I enjoy conceptualizing of different chakra realms that are all distinct and we can easily tune into. As soon as we realize that all of life is mental and that we can control PK within our chakra realms, and that these chakras are non-different from the objective world, then we can control the material world. By the way, have your chakras been treated with PK lately? Whenever one says that doing this or that leads to "good" or "bad" karma, one is already acknowledging that subjective thoughts and actions do affect the objective world. One is acknowledging the mind's ability to control the physical plane for better or worst, and what it produces in the objective world. By understanding these metaphysical concepts, we eventually attain the true independence and the most ecstatic state of *nirvana-samhadhi* in this life. Nothing is more blissful and desirable.

.

Another yogic doctrine that is easy to misinterpretation is the concept of Maya, the material illusion. According to this philosophy, everything in the material world is merely an illusion that is controlled by the mind. On a more profound structural level, this doctrine means that all of our subjective worlds are different, and that these margins of difference account for the entire material illusion. All of us have unique karma that determines our experience in life. For one person, certain things in life are easier than others and they are actually possible. For others, these same things are basically impossible in the very same world, and even hard for them to fathom doing. The material world where we now live is an illusion because we all can control the same objective world that we share in very unique ways. The difference between two people's "abilities" in the objective world makes it an illusion by nature rather than an absolute.

This difference in karmic disposition between individuals is the material illusion. One person is able to walk on water, levitate, heal the sick, levitate or fly, while another one can control the ways refrigerators function and even automobiles at a distance. So, why are some people able to perform these telekinetic feats while others are not? That all concerns the complexities of individual karma! The best kept secret is that karma can be changed through disciplinary yoga and other prescribed methods of metaphysical work.

Through engineering our subtle energy vortexes (chakras), we can apparently take control over every aspect of life. It enables us to resolve even the most complex karmic difficulties. This is primarily because the Lord God Almighty is "smaller than the smallest particle." By relying on Him to purify our chakra realms, even the most subtle forms of contamination from past lives immemorial are removed from our being. Then we can attain true independence and happiness in this world filled with misery and perilous misrepresentation. The fact that Lord Krsna as Narayana resides in the hearts of everybody evidences this inherent connection between God working within our chakras as the key to liberation from matter. The heart chakra is the gateway to the supernatural and the seat of the divine. When the heart is purified of contamination, then one becomes proportionally eligible to enter into higher planetary systems.

How do we know that there are higher planetary systems? The Vedic scriptures such as the *Bhagavad-Gita* and the Brahma Samhita all inform us that there are innumerable planets in both the material and anti-material worlds. Moreover, two American physicist Dr. Emilio Segre (born in Italy) and Dr. Owen Chamberlain (born in San Francisco, California) were awarded the Nobel Physics Prize for discovering the antiproton. They proved that matter exists in two forms, as both particles and antiparticles.

Their theory fundamentally assumes that there may be the existence of another world, which is an anti-world, composed of anti-matter. In the anti-material world, the atomic and subatomic particles spin in the opposite direction of the ones in the material world. This is consistent with what Lord Sri Krsna spoke in the *Bhagavad-Gita* about the existence of two forms of energy the material and spiritual. He also confirms that the spiritual particle is superior to the material. The anti-material world is where this superior spiritual energy originates. The anti-material particle controls matter and can never be destroyed. Everything in the material world is created and then subject to destruction at a given point. On the other hand, the anti-material particle is never created so it can not be annihilated. The *Bhagavad-Gita* confirms this, where it states that the anti-material particle "neither has birth dates or death dates...Although the material particle is annihilated, the anti-material particle is never affected." The *Bhagavad-Gita* discusses these two distinct particles in terms of energy, one being spiritual and the other material. Both the spiritual world and the material world both are inhabited with infinite planets. In fact, Lord Sri Krsna states explicitly in the *Bhagavad-Gita* that "Earth is but one grain of sand in a sandbag filled with planets."

A February 21 1960 Moscow press release reported that the prominent Russian Professor of Astronomy Boris Vorontsov-Veliaminov said that "there must be an infinite number of planets in the universe inhabited by beings endowed with reason." His position was bolstered by Professor Vladimir Alpatov who claims that some of these planets have a state of development similar to that of earth. He also said that he believes the gaseous composition of the atmosphere of Mars is quite suitable to maintain life for certain kinds of organisms. However it is crucial to note that one planet's atmosphere can not sustain life form an organism that does not have a suitable body. These claims validate information provided in the Brahma Samhita which informed us long ago that there are in innumerable number of planets and universes in existence. Furthermore, the *Brahma-Samita* states that there are a variety of planets in each of these universes.

According to the Vedanta, we are all merely transmigrating from one body to the next, from one planet to the next, from universe to the next, from one world to the next! We have the constitutional right to live on whatever planet that we please, either in the material world or the spiritual skies. The practical difference between the material and spiritual world is that the later is free from all forms of death, misery, birth and rebirth, old age, sickness and disease. On the other hand, the chief yogic scriptures reveal to us that the material world we live in right now is a place characterized by perpetual pain, constant inconveniences such as suffering, disease, old age, birth and rebirth. We can use cosmic celestial energies from the spiritual world such as PK force to create rapturous heavenly conditions right here on earth.

The Vedas further instructs us that these planets are arranged in a hierarchical systems, some being higher (heavenly) and others lower (hellish). This is also fairly in accordance with most modern religions, because the concept heaven and hell originated from the Vedas. These concepts were merely carried over into the modern religions, while other vital information was just left out. This proves that the principles of real religion can not be made up or fabricated. By definition, they come from the same source, which is why for example the Hindus, the Christians, the Mormons, and the Jahovas Witnesses all believe in "heaven" and "hell." How in the world do all of these religions have such specific things in common, unless they all come from the same source? Another thing that they all have in common is the faith in the only one God, "the Lord." Finally, they are similar in the fact that they do not know much about God's identity or personality.

Our individual Karma is what determines where the soul goes after it quits the physical body. Again, our karma can be changed through the practice of transcendental yoga. This means that we can influence what happens to us in this life and the next. Without this kind of understanding of mind over matter, the entire pursuit of transcendental and yogic knowledge is in vain, and a mere waste of time. What good is it for a man to profit the whole world with his mind over matter powers, only to loose his soul at the end? To provide further insight on this matter, Lord Sri Krsna advises in the Bhagavad-gita:

"Those who worship the demigods will take birth among the demigods; those who worship the ancestors go to the ancestors; those who worship ghost and spirits will take birth among such beings; and those who worship Me will live with Me."

Many religions promise their adherents some kind of miraculous powers by following certain guidelines. For example, Jesus Christ instructed his disciples "He that believeth on me, the works that I do shall he do also; and greater works than these shall he do." Buddhism teaches that there are six superknowledges attained through meditation. But what does the Vedic Absolute Truth tell us about attaining the supreme state? In yogic studies, we learn that the yogi who is close to being totally liberated attains "victory over matter, compounds, molecules, atoms, and ultra-atomic particles." The completely liberated yogi has even greater powers including the ability to change destiny (karma), the revelry of reality, and where he takes birth in the next life.

When everything in one's life is increasingly perfect and ideal by virtue of directly satisfying the Supreme Brahman by yogic practice, then one naturally falls deeper into trance. This results from alleviated distress on the mind and consciousness. The more stress that is alleviated form one's life, the deeper one naturally falls into trance. That is why Lord Sri Krsna, is also known as the one who takes away all distress and anxiety from His devotees.

I want to reiterate here that true-PK can be used to attain the ultimate reality and the Lord's supreme abode. By contrast, in asthanga yoga, this energy is used at some level to transport the yogi to whatever planet he desires at the moment one leaves the body. Many yogis throughout Vedic history have been able to use PK force to travel to any planet in the material world including Brahamaloka, which is the highest planetary destination in our universe. For example one demon named Ravana acquired such powers and eventually was killed by Lord Sri Krsna, for challenging His divine order, by attempting to lobby Lord Brahamaji for immortality.

The scriptures reveal to us that Lord Brahmaji resides in Brahmaloka, the highest planet in our universe. Beyond Brahmaloka, the spiritual skies begin, which is the world of innumerable spiritual planets known as the Vaikunthalokas. Only one-quarter of the Lord's creation is in the material world, while the remaining three quarters is in the spiritual skies. Many people in this age of ignorance mistakenly consider Lord Brahmaji and Lord Sri Krsna to be on the same transcendental level. Lord Brahmaji himself explicitly acknowledges in his treatise known as the Sri Brahma Samhita Chapter 5 Verse 1:

" *The Supreme Personality of Godhead is Krsna. He has an eternal, blissful, spiritual body. He is the origin of all. He has no other origin, and He is the prime cause of all causes.*"

So what about Lord Shiva? Well, it is widely recognized based on authoritative scripture that Lord Siva is a quite powerful "demigod." There is an entity known as Hari-hara who is worshiped by both devotees of Lord Vishnu and Lord Shiva. This deity confirms the Absolute Truth, as it represents how the same supreme person (Krsna) incarnated in both Vishnu and Shiva. This is consistent with the Vedas, which also teaches us that the same supreme person, Lord Sri Krsna, incarnated as both Vishnu and Shiva. However, Vishnu and Shiva are not the same kind of incarnations. Lord Shiva, as "The Destroyer" has a distinct role which is to destroy the material illusion that binds minds into the lower worlds of misery. So, Shiva worship is useful for eradicating the mentality that hinders one from making spiritual advancements towards Godhead.

Another thing that many people do not understand is that although Lord Sri Krsna is an incarnation of Vishnu pursuant to the scheme that he created. He is even to be distinguished from Vishnu. The Vedic yoga record teaches that Lord Sri Krsna created the Maha Vishnu as his immediate expansion. Then the Maha Vishnu breathed into existence innumerable worlds within the spiritual ocean. He further expanded as the Garbhodakasayi Vishnu that entered into each of the universes, for the specific purpose of creating diversity.

This is all just a part of the history of the universe, and it should not be confused with mythology. Mythology is composed of made up stories, while true, complete and comprehensive history involves real accounts from authoritative sources of information, such as the chief yogic scriptures. The history of our universe is not different. In an information age, we need to take information very seriously, especially when it comes from the most authoritative sources. This is why modern science is constantly confirming the same truths revealed by the highest gurus, sages and rishis from millions of years ago! Nobel prizes are being awarded for just confirming the same truths and verities found in the yogic world scriptures. As we will see, Charles Richet was also awarded the Nobel prize in Physiology for confirming the same basic precepts concerning Shakti energy.

The world scriptures reveal that before these two Vishnus were created by Lord Sri Krsna, He was already in existence in the spiritual skies. This entire anti-material world is free of death, rebirth, old age and sickness, which is why it is completely transcendental to lower material worlds. It is also permanent and absolute rather than illusory. The planets in the spiritual world are also stratified into a hierarchy. The scriptures indicate that the highest of these is Krsnalaloka, the abode of the Supreme Lord.

In terms of the planetary arrangement, the Lord Sri Krsna confirms in Chapter 8 Text 16 of the *Bhagavad-Gita:*

"From the highest planet in the material world down to the lowest, all are places of misery wherein repeated birth and death take place. But one who attains to My abode, O son of Kunti, never takes birth again."

Once you can see everything in life from a transcendental platform, then you have literally achieved the aim of mind over matter. All too often, students of true yoga give up before they actually see the forest for the trees and the mountains for the peaks. With a little bit more persistence, the right Guru to guide, and a connection to the highest, these neophyte yogis would have made the most powerful breakthrough and epiphany of a lifetime.

Chapter 3: Yoga and the Metaphysical Science

Every field of science rests upon certain pillars. The metaphysical or "occult" science is certainly no exception to this rule. Historically and factually, the principles of religion all come from yoga. This was explained very clearly by Lord Sri Krsna in the *Bhagavad-Gita* Chapter Four, Text One through Text Four, where Lord Sri Krsna starts out by saying "I instructed this imperishable science of yoga to the sun-god, Vivasvan, and Vivasvan instructed it to Manu, the father of mankind, and Manu in turn instructed it to Iksvaku." These were the very same exact principles of religion that passed down into all systems of yoga, the occult science, metaphysics and religion as we know it today. These are by definition the precepts of religion in the purest form, which can not be fabricated or "made up" by anybody. They are imperishable principles directly from God and His celestial heavenly hosts So does religion play a big part in the paranormal?

For your information, Vivasvan is the presiding deity or "demigod" of the sun, which is the scriptures reveal is the highest planet in our universe. The concept of administrative and executive assistants who manage the cosmic affairs is foreign to most. However, the world scriptures confirm that there are elevated personalities known as demigods who are approved by the Lord to manage the material affairs such as the rising and setting of the sun and the seasons. Lord Brahmaji for example is the chief demigod in our universe and resides on the highest planet in our universe known as *Bhamaloka*. So, he manages the affairs of our entire material world, and hence he is known as the "Grandfather." However, Lord Sri Krsna created Brahma and is worshiped by Him, so he is regarded as the "Great-grandfather." Most people take it for granted that the sun rises and sets at the exact same time everyday. They have no clue that the ancient scriptures of yoga give detailed information about this all being controlled by demigods.

The entire occult science and metaphysics was born from the royal Bhakti Yoga established by Lord Sri Krsna. This is why He is known as the Master of all Mysticism. Now, Lord Sri Krsna explains in the *Bhagavad-Gita* that the *Doctrine of the Three Gunas* is the basis of all yoga and the key to understanding our true nature. He confirms that this is all "transcendental knowledge," which liberates us from lower existence in the material world. This is the understanding that is necessary for the mind to wield the most power over matter! Therefore, *Three Gunas* stand as pillars that support all occult and metaphysical science.

At the core of this Doctrine, the highest principle is that there is a God, who is a person that we must surrender to fully before we can attain the apex of yoga. That explains why all religions acknowledge the existence of a God who we must surrender to. The main difference is that there is much more accurate information in the realm of yoga, where all religion cam from in the first instance. God's existence as an actual person with a distinct form is the *main pillar* for the entire body of "occult knowledge." In other words, God Himself is not some formless, gaseous being with no personality as some may think. The highest precepts of the occult science, mysticism and true religion teach us that He is a very real person who dwells on the highest planet in existence. This excerpt from *Sri Isopanistad* helps us to understand God's transcendental position, and the role of His innumerable demigods. This is one of my personal favorite power mantras:

"The Supreme Personality of Godhead, although fixed in His abode is more swift than the mind and can overcome all other running. The powerful demigods can not approach Him. Although in one place, He has control over those that supply the air and the rain. He surpasses all in excellence."

The highest principles of yoga also explain how this supreme person, Lord Sri Krsna, dwells within everybody's heart, as the all pervading "Supersoul".known as Paramatma. Due to the influence of time, geography and the age of ignorance (Kali), much of the modern world is unaware of these core truths about our nature and background as transmigrating souls. The validity of the Gunas as an effective mapping system for ultimate reality has been confirmed and experienced by a very long line of occultists and adepts. I also can confirm that the Doctrine of the Gunas is the most powerful road map for how to live. In fact chapter fourteen (The Three Modes of Material Nature) of the *Bhagavad-gita* clearly explains this sacred knowledge.

Understanding how the three modes of material nature function and interact is the most powerful way for using the mind to control matter. The Three Gunas are: *Sattva*, *Rajas*, and *Tamas*. They represent the elements of goodness, passion and ignorance respectively. These are the three "modes of material nature" which control every aspect of our existence in this "material world." These modes indirectly control our karma and chakras. This is another classic example of how a subjective representation of reality can be used to understand and control the objective world. The doctrine of the Gunas is the most perfect representation because it comes straight from the mouth of God, which is why it forms the very basis of the entire transcendental science. The whole material world is being controlled by these three modes. So, the highest form of mind over matter is learning to work within this mapping system.

For more detailed information regarding the Gunas, please refer to Chapter 14 entitled *The Three Modes of Material Nature* of the *Bhagavad-Gita As It Is*, by Swami Prabhupada. Many people claim to be occultists, yogis, or transcendentalist. I believe that people can only make it so high spiritually without learning the deeper principles that gave rise to these practices. According to the *Bhagavad-Gita*, we can only go so far without acknowledging the existence of Lord Sri Krsna as the supreme person, and surrounding unto Him. In the *Bhagavad-Gita*, Lord Sri Krsna clearly points out that these surrendered souls are "the highest" yogis!

So many people fail to recognize that God by His very nature actually wants us to master the principles of metaphysics, PK, mind power and the occult science. This includes knowledge of astrology, the sciences, and the properties of subtle energies. However, He can not bless us with "the highest" spiritual powers until we have surrendered unto Him. Then He reveals the most divine secrets which includes knowledge of true PK based on first hand experience. That is my personal view, which is supported by ageless information from the chief yogic literature such as Srimad

Bhagavatam.

When we use physical forms of yoga, a connection is established with specific energy fields that these postures or movements represent. This works very much like any other kind of symbolic representation or archetype. According to the concept of "structural links," there is no distance in the realm of mind between two points or intervals, where there is an effective means of making a connection between the two. By analogy, if there is six miles of distance between point A and B in the physical plane, then that distance must be traveled in order to get from one point to the next. On the other hand, in the realm of the mind, the distance is zero whenever you have an effective structural link between point A and B. That is why physical yoga can be a powerful way to link the mind with higher order energies.

Many metaphysical tools such as psychotronics operate on this same functioning principle (FP) to enable the mind to control matter. Since there is no difference between the subjective (mental) and the objective (physical) worlds, one can theoretically control the external physical world, by knowing the FP's for the mental world. Certain archetypes such as yantras (mystical symbols), mudras (mystical hand signs) and other talismans are used to make a structural connection with the specific trend energies that they represent. This is the secret to the power of these archetypes. They have been loaded with mental energies that flow through the structural links and attach to the symbol.

Over time, these symbols collect lots of "psychic energy," they become increasingly powerful and effective for manifesting on the physical what they represent in the mind. In some cultures, "healers" use blood samples, hair, a picture, clothing or nails to make a structural connection with their "targets" who may be on the other side of the world! These artifacts work well for many spiritual healers and "psychotronics operators," as they contain specific information about the patient such as their genetic code, signature, or unique appearance. Yogic postures, movements and other methods affect the mind by acting as structural links to particular trend energies. This is why metaphysical tools such as mantras are quite useful. Working with the power of sound is one of the easiest and most effective methods for tuning your mind into auspicious vibrations.

The direct knowledge of the reality that is hidden within all human beings, the universe, and the deepest levels of consciousness is the chief aim of yogic practice. When man knows that he is one with this reality through direct perception, then he is liberated from the lower worlds of illusion. The main purpose of yoga is for the individual to attain personal freedom, independence and liberation from all manners of influences. Again, on one hand we have yoga that is concerned exclusively with physical well-being and health; and on the other hand, the higher forms of yoga are designed to foster mental and spiritual perfection, mystical powers and "oneness with the divine."

Pranayama meaning breath control is a part of *Hatha-yoga* for physical vitality and it is used to release the dormant divine energy known as Kundalini. This energy is within all of us and coiled up at the base of the spine as an energy vortex. Among yogis, this Kundalini energy is regarded as the most powerful force in existence and must be handled with special care. Yogis believe that prana is inherently a part of the air, and is filtered out by special breath control techniques. They are able to exploit the air as a source of prana, which then triggers a release in the Kundalini, which is conceptually connected with "PK Force" among western scientists.

Many yogis can consciously release the Kundalini energy through regulated breathing. This leads to significant mental control over material nature. The most crucial thing to note about this energy is that it acts on its own to literally manifest anything that we want in life. It is an active creative energy that spawned the whole universe. PK energy is extremely independent and intelligent, so all that we have to do is awaken the Shaktipat (dormant Kundalini) in ourselves and develop it to the fullest extent via *bhakti-yoga*. This is exciting news for you, because this energy works very automatically, and it is up to us to understand that and to enhance it by immediately recognizing and maximizing what it brings us.

Prana itself is not Kundalini energy, but it functions to amplify the levels and functioning of Kundalini in the bio-energetic body. In Kundalini yoga, the adept is able to control the activity of this energy within the energetic body's chakras for increased control over material nature as a whole. In fact, the term transcendental literally implies "superior positioning" that enables one to control matter. Essentially, yoga involves scientific methods for empowering the higher mind to attain its fullest potential for controlling matter and energy as a whole. It enables us all to make union with the ultimate reality and personally experience spiritual life, which is real life.

Since people in our times readily accept things that they have personally experienced, yoga of all types is now more important then ever for self-realization! In prior ages, stories from others regarding their experiences were readily accepted and believed by most, but nowadays we all demand as much tangible proof as possible. It has reached the point where many wont believe in anything that they have not experienced for themselves. Even despite this first hand experience with the supernatural, many people still resist it to the fullest. However, personal experiences always give rise to some spiritual advancement.

In the schools of Eastern mysticism, it is well known that these personal experiences begin after the awakening of Kundalini energy. One crucial aim of this manuscript is to give readers the tools for triggering their own spiritual breakthroughs, awakenings and experiences that can not be ignored. Kundalini energy is essentially Shakti, which is the power that leads us back to God! There are many ways to trigger an awakening of Kundalini. Unfortunately, many material scientists today have a narrow clinical view of this force. So, they lack complete information regarding Kundalini, and thus regard it as an ordinary material energy, rather than cosmic by its nature.

In the East, where this energy and its verities have been analyzed since the remotest times, the primary authorities on the subject are the scriptures of the Vedanta and Shaivism. In fact, the term Kundalini originated from these scriptures, where it is called "Divine consciousness." The energy is omniscient and its properties and FP's are not the subject of physics, biology, chemistry, psychology, or any of the material sciences. The sacred yogic scriptures confirm that the main purpose of this energy is to guide us all back to God. Any incidental effects such as typical "psi phenomenon" are only bi-products of Kundalini and potential distractions. These psi effects are great for helping us understand the reality of Kundalini via personal experience. This energy is really Lord Sri Krsna (God) manifesting through His potencies and multifarious energies. It leads us back to the original transcendental plane of perfection and enlightenment.

The sages of India worship this energy as the Divine Mother Shakti, the consort of Lord Shiva and also as Laxmi who is the consort of Lord Vishnu . It is the active feminine aspect of the Supreme Brahman. Indeed it is the highest and most powerful creative energy! In every culture, this energy is acknowledged in some form. In China, it is associated with Chi, while in Japan it is related to Ki, and among the Westerners it is connected with the concept of "life energy." Another term for Kundalini derived from the ancient *Shaivite* scriptures is Chiti, meaning "universal consciousness."

Again, Kundalini is a highly independent cosmic energy that creates everything on its own volition, without any reliance on any outside agencies. It is the cosmic force that manifests into this multi-faceted universe. Many exercises and other yogic methods have been continuously developed over time for awakening this supreme force within us all. By utilizing these prescribed methods to stimulate this power within, we automatically trigger a boost in telekinetic and mind over matter potential. This is discussed more extensively in the later chapter on "telekinetic triggers."

Again, true-yoga is the essence of real-religion, it is unlimited, and there are many different types used for myriad purposes. *Hatha-yoga* gives one mastery over breath which fosters control over the physical body and vitality. Laya, in the term *laya-yoga* refers to 'mind-control' and it is that part of yogic science concerned primarily with the method of achieving mastery over the mind and will power. That is especially important in terms of controlling PK, because PK is directly controlled by our will power. That is why *laya-yoga* is known to create the highest levels of independence and freedom from the material body, which makes us suspended in bliss and spiritual ecstasy. Laya leaves the mind suspended in a blissful state, as the PK is under more unconscious control, which alleviates pressure on the conscious mind.

While in Bhakti Yoga, one-pointedness of mind is achieved by yogic concentration on an object of Divine Love, in Shakti Yoga a "yogically equivalent" result is fostered through focusing on Divine Power as Shakti. Thus, *shakti-yoga* involves practices, principles, methods and processes for mastering the ability to enhance and control Divine Power in our lives! Here, we are referring to the same energy that yogis throughout history have used develop their "telekinetic" powers. These powers may include levitation, bi-location, inter-dimensional travel, teleportation, telepathy, ESP, and weather control. Although Eastern and Western "scientist" view this energy in different contexts, both perspectives enable us to better understand it.

By merely contemplating and studying various forms of transcendental yoga, one becomes spiritually purified and advanced. My greatest breakthroughs in mysticism only occurred as a result of engaging my mind in transcendental subject matter. I started out practicing Bhakti Yoga, which eventually led to a total restructuring of my Karma. Much of this spiritual progress is made possible by the grace of a Guru who is empowered to renew our divine consciousness. Frankly, I consider the Guru-disciple relationship as one of the most important aspects of this whole life. Lord Sri Krsna Himself, the creator of all, values guru-disciple relations and always charges it with great spiritual power.

There is Jewish DNA in India, which substantiates the fact that Jews settled down there, especially in the region of Kashmir. Many genetic tests have been carried out involving the Bene Israel Jews from Alibag India. These studies validate stories from the Indians that Jews traveled to and settled in India. For the sake of your understanding, great saints are never cremated. Only the common man or woman is cremated, but yogi's, saints and pure devotees of God are not. It is understood that these great souls enter into an elevated and enlightened state of consciousness before proceeding to the spiritual word. This consciousness is called "samadhi." Hence, their bodies are preserved in what many call a tomb, but we call (transcendental) samadhi. In fact many great saints including Moses, Aaron, Solomon and Jesus all have samadhi's in Kashmir. It is a fact that you can visit some of them even today! This arrangement allows for everyone to continue reaping benefit from them. Many of you have heard about miracles happening when someone touched a sacred garment worn by a saint, visited their 'tomb' (samadhi), prayed in their 'presence,' or something else. Either an obvious external miracle is experienced or deeper karmic spiritual changes occur.

When great yogis are in samadhi, even when their bodies are buried, they continue existing in a transcendental position. There are numerous classic reports of yogis' being buried in trance and exhumed in good condition many hours later. A yogi can stay alive in a transcendental state even if buried not only for many days but for many years! Paramahansa Yoganada is a classic example of how a master yogi's body can remain preserved and in good condition even after passing away. This is partially attributed to the fact that the yogis have been working so closely with anti matter, which neutralizes certain material processes. More about this can be read in Srimad Bhagavatam, 7.3.18 .

So , why is it like pulling wisdom teeth to get people to understand that Jesus traveled to and retired in India? Most of his entire life is not even accounted for in the Bible. This disbelief is probably caused by fundamentalist indoctrination. Similarly, people can not fathom Jesus meditating in a lotus position, worshipping Lord Jagannatha (Krishna) or reading the Vedic scriptures. True disciples of Christ do not question his activities that are on record only because it is something new to them. His most intelligent followers will do their "due diligence," and embrace the truth as soon as they find it.

Christ and his disciples converged in Jerusalem to carry out his instructions and spread his message around the world. Wherever they went the message was the same: To glorify the Holy Names of God, pray to "the Father," and to seek the face of God the Father (Krishna) for salvation. So they divided many countries up between themselves. Interestingly enough, "Doubting Thomas" was specifically dispatched to India.

This is a well accepted fact even by Christians today. Saint Thomas is known to have been many places in India and his presence and writings are still acknowledged by the people. Based on a wealth of evidence, many people contend that Kashmir, India is the Promised Land that Jesus referred to. It is common knowledge that ten lost tribes of Israel migrated down to Afghanistan and Kashmir, India. Kashmir was a much more friendly environment for the Jewish people. Christ was the Messiah and his specific mission from God/Krishna was to save the Jewish people and lead them to the Promised Land.

India is just one of the many nations and scriptures that refer to Lord Jesus Christ, In the ancient Purana section called the Bhavisya (pronounced Bhavishya) Purana, it is clearly stated that Jesus was in India). Even if one does not believe the *Bhavisya Purana* as truth, there is a wealth of other evidence proving that Jesus traveled to many lands that are not recorded within the Bible; and that he also continued his mission in India. More evidence is provided in the *Bhavisya Purana* regarding his worship of Lord Jagannatha in the Jagannatha Puri temple, India.

His mission was that of the Messiah and savior of the Jews. He was to stop the sales of animals in the temples and meat eating of the people (as well as also giving instructions on illicit sex). Then, to give them higher knowledge, to deliver them to the Holy Land of India, until gradually they might be fortunate enough to open up and hear exactly who God ss: Lord Sri Krsna. Jesus was their Messiah and he was a Vaishnava devotee. Many people wonder why we do not see Christ on record directly preaching about Krishna. It is certainly not because he did not accept Krishna as God, but because the masses were not advanced enough to take heed to the few enlightened ones.

The expanded   consciousness that we experience by practicing royal yoga   begins automatically working in our lives and gradually purifies all of our chakras. That is indeed the highest and most effective form of "self-help." It marks the beginning of real-life for many, because the energy can make anything happen for us. There are unlimited ways for the Guru to awaken this divine consciousness in disciples. In many cases, PK phenomenon begins or increase dramatically almost immediately after the Guru emerges in the disciple's life. For example, many disciples of Satiya Sai Baba constantly report the most amazing miracles in their environment shortly after accepting him as their Guru. You only must up to accepting the grace of the Guru, worship the Guru as you worship God, and receive him as God's divine representative on Earth.

According to Sri Yukteswar, the Guru of Paramahansa Yogananda, "neither the East nor the West will flourish without the pervasive practice of disciplinary yoga." The easiest most sublime way to make progress in spirituality and disciplinary yoga is through the grace of a Divine Guru. The purpose of a Guru is to shine like the sun, to illuminate and vanquish darkness of delusion! The Guru-disciple relationship should be promoted by the society as a whole and pervasively understood. I believe that the Guru should be sought from the time of our birth, which is the case in many cultures.

Many people in the world simply do not know that it is necessary to have a Guru guide your steps. My life would be unbearably destructive without the influence of my Gurus. The most unfortunate souls are under the false impression that a Guru can be supplanted with other things. This special arrangement by the Supreme Creator can lead to the cultivation of strong telekinetic potential, as the Guru has more hands-on experience to reveal these secrets powers to the disciple. The guru can literally bless the disciple with control over the divine kundalini energy. He can also initiate the disciple, and awaken the kundalini at will through a mere touch, a stare, an incantation, or a thought; this is known as *Shaktipat Diksha.*

My PK powers were actually triggered, amplified, and enhanced by my Austrian Guru Sri Prananand, who just happened to be a biophysicist. Interestingly enough, he was the only person who could help me to make sense of the most mysterious aspects of my life. Many people told me that they would never be able to handle living with the kind of miracles and psi phenomenon I experienced constantly after meeting my Guru without eventually losing their minds. It is not necessary for anybody to loose their minds, because there are many gracious gurus on the planet right now such as myself, who are waiting to help people with self realization!

Without the divine influence and involvement of my Gurus, I would be stuck in utter confusion regarding my own true nature, power and potential. I am almost afraid to think of what my life would be like right now without the influence of my God-sent Gurus. Many people around the world are totally unfamiliar with the critical concept of the guru-disciple relationship, so I admonish everybody to learn more about its value and to find your Guru. Those who are oblivious of this essential yogic precept go through life taking for granted that single most valuable person when they come around. However, this is the most critical and sacred relationship in our entire lives, and should never be taken for granted! If Arjuna did not accept the Grace of his Guru, Lord Sri Krsna on the battlefield of Kuruksetra, things would have turned out much differently. Instead, Arjuna absorbed what Lord Sri Krsna was teaching him like a sponge, with no resistance and total submission. This is the best example of how disciples are to surrender unto their Gurus.

Based on one's karma, one may only have very limited chances in a lifetime to cultivate this relationship. This is why the yogic scriptures advise us to always carry a loving disposition and to cultivate friendship. If we are not amicable and receptive to the gurus when they come around, then they can not help us out of the material mire. Part of the power in this relationship comes from the fact that it helps us to 'survive" by stimulating the root chakra. This chakra center is specifically connected with friendship, brotherhood, comradery, and community. These are a major aspects of being "grounded" and surviving as humans.

There are two kind of Gurus that must be distinguished: The *Siksa-guru is* one that initiates us into general and basic metaphysical matters. One the other hand, the Diksha Guru is one who performs the process of Shaktipat Diksha that awakens our dormant kundalini. The specific role of the Diksha Guru is to awaken this divine kundalini energy, by spiritually initiating the disciple into Krsna Consciousness. Prabhupada states:

"One should take initiation from a bonafide spiritual master coming in the disciplic succession, who is authorized by his predecessor spiritual master. This is called diksa-vidhana." (Srimad-Bhagavatam, 4.8.54, purport)

Note that both of these Gurus are considered God's worshipable divine representatives on earth. In this day and age, without having a Guru to guide one in the right direction, it becomes increasingly difficult for students of yoga, the occult sciences and metaphysics to actually make the connection with the very forces they seek to understand and control. In this age of *Kali-yuga*, the time of great despair, peril, darkness and ignorance, the Guru-disciple relationship is more critical than ever.

Chapter 4 : Spiritualistic Mediums and Early PK Research

Innovative scientific technology has been used, since the incipient phases of psi research and PK experimentation. We can not escape the influence of technology on any modern discovery or breakthrough. Naturally, the next step beyond the discovery of a force such as PK is the development of increasingly advanced, sophisticated and powerful apparatus for testing and working with the energy. Many PK researchers from various disciplines and professional backgrounds have made phenomenal discoveries. These include engineers, biologists, physicists, psychiatrists and physiologists.

The Society of Psychical Research was established in 1882 and pioneered many psi experiments, in response to spontaneous reports of paranormal activity. Prior to its establishment, nearly all recorded cases of PK involved seance settings and isolated poltergeist activities within homes. As these claims were consistently observed, reported, and confirmed by eye witnesses, some of the world's leading scientists began taking a much closer look. Since then, many controlled experiments have been conducted in seance settings to more closely examine this force in action. Researchers consistently have confirmed things happening during the seances that are totally inexplicable under conventional scientific thought. In many cases, tables suddenly turned or tipped over, while other pieces of furniture moved and levitated during seances. In other cases, phantom figures appeared out of nowhere.

The "sitters" who attended the seances were often physically touched by these apparitional forms. In many instances, the effects of PK lingered in the seance room well after it was over. That is known as the "linger-effect" among PK researchers. By the way, it is hard to overlook the semantic similarities between the terms *seance* and *science*. The entire field of psi was born out of these controlled seance studies involving all forms of PK. Based on numerous findings and their implications, PK is compelling more attention then any other area of parapsychology.

In considering research, we must address a number of issues and difficulties at the outset. First off, what is research? When does it conclusively produce a finding? There are so many different types of research, which lead to similar problems. For example, all of the following approaches to research create problems when trying to specify a finding, in terms of their reliability and validity: Case studies; public opinion polls; field surveys; questionnaires; formal tests connected with behavioral measures; and experiments where all relevant variables are controlled, except for the independent variables manipulated by the experimenter. All of these forms of research present issues in being sufficiently detailed, with adequate information to justify a conclusive finding. However, they have all past the rigorous test of time as useful ways of studying an experience, process or phenomenon.

In the field of psychology, various research methods are used such as naturalistic observations, research reports produced by anthropologists and sociologists. These are typically very subjective, informal, and lack the reliability and control of laboratory research. However, they are still classified as research that can produce valid findings.

As wee can see, controlled laboratory experiments are not the only acceptable form of scientific research. However, many people give it far more weight than it warrants. Empirical observations under the right conditions may be just as "reliable" and "valid" as any other form of research, and even more trustworthy in cases where there are multiple eye witness! Thus, the vast majority of people make the mistake of ignoring this kind of hard evidence to their own detriment. Empirical research can even be more valuable than laboratory experiences, depending on the nature of the experience. If we carelessly discard the experiences and observations involved with empirical research, then life itself is a waste.

The best way to resolve this issue is to recognize that all forms of research can be equally valid and effective in yielding evidence. In the case of my discoveries with the FP, both empirical and controlled research approaches have been used to confirm its existence. All forms of research should be equally scrutinized and criticized based on methodology and conditions. Some research findings gathered in participant observation studies should be treated with equal weight as those conduced in laboratories under experimental conditions. Research is only as good as the evidence that it provides, and eye-witness testimonies are always regarded as a form of evidence. This is even the case within the law of evidence used in courts.

If we acknowledge detailed reports validated by bonafide spiritual masters and authorities, accounts of PK could be traced back to the remotest of times. In fact, the Mahabharata, the Ramayana and even the Bible are filled with classic examples of the limitless powers and potential of God and the human mind. Clearly, the idea that the human mind controls matter is nothing new. However, it was not until the nineteenth century in England that PK was first investigated experimentally by William Crooks, a chemist working with the famous medium D.D. Home. Crookes performed experiments on Home using ingenious weighing apparatus that actually measured energy proceeding from his hands. These experiments established that Home had mastered a new form of energy they labeled "psychic force." During these experiments, Home levitated in good lighting and with no props.

Home was known for elongating his body by paranormal means, and for handling burning coals without incurring any injuries. He even convinced others to handle the coals who also were uninjured. One of his most notorious feats was immunity to fire, and unlike other mediums, he rarely ever conducted his seances in the dark. Home and his experimenters would sit around a table in quite strong lighting. First, he would enter into a deep trance, and then a variety of PK phenomenon would begin happening. Tables tipped while furniture levitated. He materialized apparitional forms in the seance rooms, produced psychic lights, and channeled messages from dead spirits.

Home was also well known for his ability to activate an accordion instrument without even touching it. One of his strongest supporters was the Englishman, Lord Adare, who served as his companion in the late 1860's. Adare published one of the most significant works on PK ever written entitled *Experiences with D.D. Home*. In this volume, he reported that during certain seances, there were cold currents out of nowhere, strong vibrations and rapping noises. Home caused hands to appear during one seance that touched and seized many of the sitters who were present. Strange sounds were witnessed by all of the sitters at this seance, which came from a large writing table. According to Adare, Home's PK did not only occur during the seances. It lingered in the room well after the seance was over.

William Crookes was one of the most prominent scientists in Great Britain during his time. He was a member of the Royal Society and invented many spectacular scientific devices. Initially, he was quite skeptical about the paranormal, PK and spiritualism. However, his doubt was destroyed after conducting some of the most ingenious PK experiments to date with D.D. Home. After studying Home closely, Crooks postulated that the human body houses a force that modern science has somehow overlooked. Incidentally, this is precisely what the Vedic scriptures teach us about the nature of kundalini. Crooks was determined to measure this force in his experiments with Home, which were published in the July 1871 edition of the *Quarterly Journal of Science*.

Crookes began one experiment with Home by having him activate a piano accordion instrument without touching it. He placed the instrument into a protective cage as an experimental control, to hinder it from being touched by anybody. The tests were conducted in a laboratory and Home was immediately successful in activating the accordion. In fact, it produced many sounds even though Home had no way at all of touching the keyboard. The accordion eventually floated in the cage while continuing to play music.

In another experiment with Home, Crooks constructed a special weighing apparatus built from a thirty-six inch mahogany board.

One end of the board was bolted onto a table. The other end extended outward from the table by two feet, and it was connected to a cable that ran to an overhead spring-balance. Under ordinary conditions without any paranormal activity, applying pressure to the end of the board that was bolted to the table would not register any weight on the overhead spring balance. However, by applying any degree of pressure on the end of the board extending away from the table, the spring-balance overhead would naturally register that amount of weight.

For the experiment, Crooks instructed Home to apply his PK to the end of the board that was bolted to the table. This experiment was designed to determine if Home could cause the spring balance to register weight by touching the end of the board bolted to the table. Interestingly enough, Home succeeded easily at causing the balance to register up to seven pounds of weight by merely touching the bolted end of the board with his finger. The pressure created by his PK caused the opposite end of the board to bend downward. During this test, Home was sitting down quite relaxed and only lightly touching the board. Crooks tested the apparatus with his full body weight by standing on the end of the board that was bolted to the table; the very same end that Home touched with his finger to register weight. Even by standing on it, Crooks was only able to create a measurement of no more than two pounds!

Although Crooks was convinced of the existence of PK because of these experiments, he wanted to conduct further confirmatory tests. I certainly can relate to his critical and skeptical feeling because even after I was firmly convinced of the existence of the FP, I had to confirm my belief with further experimentation. Like Crooks, I was not at all disappointed in my findings. Crooks published an article in the October 1871 edition of the *Quarter Journal of Science*, where he substantiated the pilot experiments with Home and rebutted criticisms of his methodology. He then successfully replicated these studies under even more stringent testing conditions.

In follow up experiments, Crooks wanted to test Home using a variation of the mahogany-board setup. This time he wanted Home having as little contact with the board as possible. So, he invented a new setup that was a modification of the mahogany-board apparatus initially used. In these experiments, Home never touched the board and the same weighing method was used with the overhead springboard balance. In one trial, Crooks placed a glass of water on the end of the board that was bolted to the table. He then instructed Home to merely place a finger in the water and project his PK onto the board. This experiment was extremely successful, even though Home made no direct contact with board itself.

An immense amount of PK was somehow applied to the apparatus. Crookes reported that the end of the board extending from the table actually bent down for about 10 seconds, and then it descended even further. The mahogany board then rose back to its original position, and gradually sunk again for another 17 seconds, where it stayed until the experiment was over. It eventually returned back to its original position. According to Crookes, the strongest amount of PK pressure that Home applied to the board recorded during this experiment was equivalent to a weight of "5,000 grains of sand."

Ultimately, Crooks removed Home from having any contact with the apparatus. Still, he was able to affect the weighing device, even while standing up to three feet away from it. Crooks reported these experiments in the January 1874 issue of the *Quarterly Journal of Science*. His report also described many other arbitrary and spontaneous telekinetic effects observed in Home's presence. This included the movement of large objects, loud raps, levitation, materializations of phantom limbs and other forms.

Even in light of this priceless PK research, and the studies involving PK of many other scientists, organized science during the Victorian Era largely ignored it. However, scientists all over the world started paying much closer attention to the subject of PK after the emergence of Eusapia Palladino from Bari, Italy during the 1890's. As a young child, many telekinetic phenomenon were noticed in her environment. Palladino was initially investigated as a teenager by scientists and psychic investigators. Later she was studied by the

Director of the Institute General Psychologique in Paris between 1893 to 1894.

Initially her main ability was micro-PK, but after working under the tutelage of the prominent Italian spiritualist, Signor Damiani, her abilities greatly expanded. She is known for producing a variety telekinetic effects including: table movements; levitations; paranormal effects on clothing and curtains in the seance room; the paranormal production of music from instruments; triggering cold winds; created mysterious voices in the room; manifesting apparitional forms and much more. She worked closely with some of the world's most prominent scientists in her time including the Nobel Laureate in Physiology and Medicine Charles Richet. He was a well respected physiology professor from Paris who closely studied psychic phenomenon in seance settings. He was firmly convinced many times while in Palliadino's presence that her telekinetic powers were genuine and real.

A very extreme case happened when Richet witnessed Palladino move tables and displace many other objects in the seance room. On time Richet reported that in good lighting a table floated on its own, while one of the investigators looked underneath and confirmed that no one was touching it, and other observers watched it from above. After studying metaphysical phenomenon of all sorts, Richet concluded that "the human personality has both material and psychological powers that we do not know. In our present state of knowledge we are not in a position to know." In 1908, the Society for Psychical Research sent out some of its brightest and most skilled investigators to meet with Palladino in Naples, Italy.

They produced an extensive report delineating 470 psychic effects that none of them could explain. During these feats, Palladino experienced a number of interesting physical reactions such as violent bodily jerking, and even once had an orgasm out of nowhere during a test. This massive release of energy apparently triggered quite dramatic PK effects. I think that these symptoms could have been clear signs of some kind of demonic possession caused by her working with certain malevolent spirits! That kind of spiritual activity is expressly discouraged within the word of God.

Palladino was tied down during all of these experiments to control her movements. Despite these stringent experimental controls, she still was able to levitate household objects using her PK. She moved large pieces of furniture around the room, and made floating hands appear out of nowhere that touched people and even seized them. An international team of researchers and scientists eventually invited her to The Milan Commission for several in depth experiments. Again, during these studies she somehow caused disembodied hands to float around the room and even touch many of the observers.

Palladino claimed that her "fluidic-double" was causing these PK effects to happen. This is interesting to compare with traditions in both the East and Western occultism, which both maintain that each person possesses a secondary non-physical "subtle body." Many Western scientists know that this body image is encoded into the homonucleus of the brain. Among the Egyptians, this body is known as Ka, while in schools yoga we refer to it as the pranic body. In esoteric circles it is referred to as the *etheric body*. The common thread among all of these traditions is that this "body" is composed of more subtle matter than its physical counterpart. By developing this body and its energy centers (the chakras), one attains higher faculties for perceiving and knowing ultimate reality and the absolute truth..

The National Laboratory for Psychical Research was founded in London by Harry Price a prominent British scientist, parapsychologist and ghost-hunter. Price was notorious for his extensive PK experiments in the 1920's, which involved two subjects from Austria and one from England. He was a professor, a philosopher and an expert magician who was skilled in recognizing mediumistic fraud during PK research. One day while riding on a train between London and his home in Pulborough, Price fortuitously encountered Stella Crenshaw, a beautiful young woman who was riding in his same cabin.

As they began discussing psychical research, Stella mentioned her persistent experiences and symptoms of PK that she could not ignore. These included many kinds of raps, cold breezes, displacement of objects and other paranormal effects in her environment. Initially, Stella had no idea that Price was England's leading psychical researcher and parapsychologist. Ironically , she quickly became his most valuable PK research subject.

Price conducted these experiments in his private laboratory and employed many different devices including a self-registering thermometer on the wall which was monitored by a camera. Any slight temperature shift in the laboratory was photographed. During these seance experiments, all doors remained locked and everyone present was seated around a table as an experimental control. The thermometer consistently registered degrees much lower than the normal temperature during the experiments.

Price used a variety of apparatus to observe the effects of the PK force. One measurement device he used was an electrical pressure switch mounted inside of a cup. It was placed on a table that sometimes levitated during seances. This device was connected to an external light, which was activated by the pressure switch. Price also invented a special seance table to monitor Stella's PK that preclude any cheating. Prior to this invention, PK researchers within seance experiments would simply check the hands and feet of the mediums whenever an object in the room moved. Since, Price felt that there was a better and more scientifically reliable way of testing PK, he constructed this special table. It was quite small with a trap door cut in the top. This trap laid flat down with no handle, so that it could not be opened from the top. The only way to open it was by pushing on the underside of the table. Price then placed wire gauze around the legs of the table which extended towards the ground. A board was then placed on the wire setup and this formed a large compartment. He placed musical instruments inside the secured compartment to test if Stella could effect them with her PK.

Price also used a "shadow apparatus" for recording any ghost-like figures that materialized during seances. This handy device was composed of a lense that projected a straight light several feet onto a viewing screen. It was designed to record and observe any materialized or partially materialized forms crossing the beam. At least on one occasion, such a form was observed during the seance with Stella. However, during research it was determined that she could only produce these effects while in a state of trance or hypnosis, and while under the influence of her separate personality. While in this altered state of consciousness, she was able to levitate and move small objects with intense focus, create temperature fluctuations of more than twenty degrees and levitate herself.

Stella was also known for activating the "telekinetiscope," which is still regarded as one of the most ingenious devices ever used for PK experimentation. Price invented this contraption from a bell jar fixed on a metal base. A telegraph-type key was placed within the jar that would signal the experimenters if depressed, by setting off a light or a bell. The key was shielded by a bubble blown around it. To activate the telekinetiscope, Stella's PK would need to enter the jar, go through the bubble without popping it and then generate enough force to depress the key. It was impossible to trigger or activate the telekinetiscope in any other way.

Stella submitted to thirteen seance tests in Price's laboratory. Most importantly, these experiments were all specially designed to preclude mediumistic fraud. During the first experiment, she managed to levitate two tables, but did not show any signs of entering trance to produce these effects. The second seance was much more dramatic. Stella fell deep into a trance, the table levitated six times and the temperature dropped by roughly 12 degrees! Fortunately, Price setup temperature gauges that were closely monitored , so that nobody could argue that the cold draft that pervaded the room was hallucinatory. Price closely recorded the temperature changes and photographed all of them. This is quite similar to the temperature changes that were observed during my own PK research with the FP.

During the third experiment, the most spectacular PK effects happened. According to Price, the table levitated several times and remained in the air for many seconds. At one point, it even rose well above the heads of everybody sitting. Two of the legs then broke away from the table, which made a loud sound. The whole table eventually snapped suddenly and the top broke into two pieces. At the same time, the legs that remained on the table crumbled up. Price said that the entire table was "reduced to what is little more than matchwood."

The fourth seance experiment was no less remarkable, and Stella showed even more symptoms of trance. In her altered states of consciousness, she manifested both ESP and PK capabilities. She somehow was able to generate telekinetic lights in the seance room, out of nowhere. During this experiment, the table pivoted up on two legs so securely that it could not be pushed back down to the floor by anybody who attempted!

At one point during the experiments, a huge 16-inch sprig of lilac in full bloom fell right into the seance room out of nowhere. After participating in thirteen seance experiments and marrying Price, Stella retired from her participation in psychic investigation. She found that it was emotionally taxing, too stressful, physically difficult, and that it disrupted her whole life. I have also found that PK research and experimentation causes me to feel very anxious, tense, emotionally uneasy and physically drained. This is why I only experiment with their PK in order to run tests for proof.

Stella's experiments with Price are regarded as the most important in the history of psychic research for many reasons; primarily because they were specifically designed to preclude fraud. Prior to the research that Price performed, many parapsychologists went through extreme measures to ensure experimental control at all times, and to prevent mediumistic fraud. Researchers needed to preclude "PK agents" (research subjects) from using any slight of hand techniques, foreign props, and materials/substances to create visual impressions.

Price also worked closely with Wili and Rudi Scheider of Bramau, Austria during the 1920's in his PK research. During adolescence, both of the Austrian brothers displayed strong telekinetic powers. Initially, Willi ,the older brother, was trained by a prominent German pathologist, the Baron Dr. Albert von Schrenck-Notzing. Eventually, he worked with both brothers in developing their PK abilities. Like my Austrian Guru has instructed me, Dr. Albert von Schrenck-Notzing believed that the two brother's powers could be enhanced and developed further. So, he faithfully served as their mentor/Guru to prepare them for scientific research studies.

At first the brothers only performed the seances for their family. Typically, the sitters and the mediums sat around a table in a circle, while many objects were placed strategically around the room. Willi was the main medium and his brother did not even attend the seances until much later. During experiments, Willi was covered in luminous pins as an experimental control to in the dark seance rooms, so that his body could be monitored. Even with very severe experimental controls used, he was still able to manifest telekinesis, materialization phenomenon, and move objects placed in completely sealed cages were moved.

In 1922, Willi was formally tested by Price and Dr. Eric Dingwall who was SPR's research officer. Price and Dingwall both traveled to Germany to test Willi in three seance experiments. The conditions during these trials were strictly controlled, lots of PK activity was observed and recorded. For example, a musical box began playing on and off, and it actually wound itself up. Price reported that a hand-like figure picked up his handkerchief from his pocket several times during this experiment. All of the telekinetic effects occurred at a distance several feet away from Willi. Loud raps were heard inside a cabinet, which the researchers considered a phenomenal manifestation of PK. All of this activity was observed under good lighting conditions.

Price and Rudi also worked together experimentally in April of 1926. He took all measures to ensure that Rudi could not fake any

PK feats. Rudi produced extraordinary effects during the experiments including cold breezes, materialized hands, and a variety of rapping sounds. Based on what happened, many other scientists, researchers and investigators were prompted to study Rudi. He eventually became one of the most famous and controversial mediums in the world. This controversy compelled the attention of several world renown investigators such as Harry Price, Karl Krall, Fritz Grunewald, Schrenck-Notzing and many others.. Prior techniques for controlling the medium, such as hand control, and outlining the medium's body with luminous pins were not secure enough to satisfy the skeptics. So, Price ultimately devised another ingenious control system. Rudi participated in experiments using this new system in 1929. The system Price created this time was composed of many electrical circuits connected to the medium. The hands were locked in special gloves, and the feet were placed on metal inductors.

These circuits were connected to a display board, with many lights corresponding to each circuit. This setup prevented mediums from escaping experimental control. Lights would go out on the display board, if control was broken by moving a hand or foot. The mediums were supposed to remain totally still. The investigators would immediately know if the subject evaded control, as soon as he moved a body part. In the experiments with Rudi using these devices, Price required all the sitters at the seance to connect to the machine for complete experimental control, and they were all perfectly monitored.

This experimental control device was used in all of the experiments that Price conducted with Rudi. Typically the experiments began with Rudi entering into an altered state of consciousness or "trance." He would then become possessed by another spirit or personality named Olga. Even with all of the controls instituted by Price, Rudi displayed phenomenal telekinetic effects. For example, the seance table was dislocated, curtains suddenly and violently moved by themselves, phantom hands materialized and were observed, random body parts such as fingers and arms were seen floating.

According to the reports, there was a paper waste basket in the seance room that was lifted by a phantom hand, and even hurled at the sitters at one point. Again in this trial we witness a "trade off effect" where Rudi is possessed by a foreign spirit personality in exchange for powerful telekinetic abilities. If we have a choice of who to bargain with for our PK powers, then we had better opt to trade with the Supreme Personality of Godhead Lord Sri Krsna, for the highest powers imaginable. The resulting mind state is not demonic possession, multiple personality disorders, schizophrenic delusion and physical punishment. Instead, we receive the most sublime and transcendental gift of *Samadhi*. It is obvious by now that *Samadhi* is the plane where we observe the most transcendental telekinetic effects.

After working successfully with Price, Rudi was involved with several ingenious tests developed by Dr. Eugene Osty. He was a French physician from the Institute Metapsychique in Paris in 1930. Osty was also chiefly concerned with precluding fraud during these tests and took all measures to do so. His research design lead to a fascinating discovery in the field of PK. In terms of my discovery, the FP, it is crucial to note that the possibility of fraud is automatically eliminated because there is no way to fraudulently control refrigerators.

Osty constructed a device in the experimental room that projected an inferred beam. The beam acted as a guard to separate Rudi from the objects that he was trying to affect by his PK. For example, if he tried to grab an object and cast it about, in order to mimic a PK affect, the fraud would immediately be detected , as soon as his hand penetrated the beam. This disruption in the beam would trigger a camera and a photo would be taken of the research subject.

Under controlled testing conditions, Osty observed a grey fog which pushed and moved the seance table around. On two occasions the inferred device was triggered, and the camera flashed indicating that something had penetrated the beam. When the photos were developed, it was apparent that Rudi's hands were under experimental control. Osty finally recognized that a force was leaving Rudi's body, which while normally invisible to the eye had sufficient properties to absorb 30 percent of the beam and set off the cameras.

We should not forget that "psychokinesis" is only a label for a phenomenon. However, it is not a full blown explanation for it. Continental European researchers have many ways of labeling PK. For example, they consider any unexplained physical manifestation such as motion at a distance "telekinesis." On the other hand, when this energy became a material substance it was termed "ectoplasm." All of these are only labels but not explanations of anything.

It is critical to note that as soon as the mainstream science concedes that they do not know of the nature of this superior or "transcendental" form of energy, the "transcendental science" of yoga is automatically triggered and pulled in to explain it. Actually, the transcendental yogic sciences are much more authoritative and concrete in their positions regarding the nature and explanations for PK. One main purpose of this book is to draw critical correlations between this sacred science and the modern science of psi to help the reader grasp the Absolute Truth.

The sky is certainly the limit for those who understand the nature and functioning principles of true-PK. For example, PK is very much involved with Astral Projection and controlling it *at will*. However, until now most people had no clue that there was any connection between them. By learning to control your levels of PK, astral projection becomes second nature and you can go all over the place with ease. You can visit relatives and friends, travel to distant worlds an defiantly perform the "impossible" through the agency of telekinetic force. It is literally your ticket to the supernatural worlds, and the realm of the paranormal.

In another test, Dr. Osty hooked up a bell device to the same infrared setup instead of connecting it to the cameras. He wanted to see how long the energy would manipulate the bell. Rudi's PK consistently rang the bell for periods of more than one minute. Prompted by this new discovery, Dr. Osty decided to revise the infrared projection even further. He modified it so that a recording could be made of the precise oscillations of the beam just as Rudi's PK penetrated it.

By using this complex design, he was not only able to gauge the duration of the PK effect, it also enabled him to record the level of density and volume as the PK force interrupted the beam. His intent was to measure the energy in different ways for analysis. Osty found that Rudi's PK did oscillate, while it interacted with the beam. However, the investigator made one further discovery about Rudi's PK. Rudi always hyperventilated during his sessions. Sometimes he would breath 120 to 300 times per minute. The PK oscillations were always found to be exact double that of his respiration rate.

This establishes a definite correlation between the PK and the breath, which supports *pranayama* (breath control) theories within yoga. In *Hatha-yoga*, pranayama is used to affect the divine kundalini, which is directly tied into telekinetic activity. It also supports my belief that by mentally connecting with lower spirits for mediumistic purposes, the individual can be subjected to many undesirable repercussions. Therefore, the ideal way to amplify PK energy for testing purposes is to engage in yoga or meditation.

In the Soviet Union, PK is more heavily researched than any other nation in the world. The Russian scientists are well known for their profound understanding and strong interest in all realms of psi research, and particularly in PK Modern Russian parapsychologists consider PK as a biological force which they call "bioplasma." Many Soviet researchers believe that bioplasma can leave the human body and create a number of telekinetic effects, or produce a duplicate body within the physical body called the "bioplasmic body." This is conceptually very similar to what the Eastern yogic scriptures of Shaivism teach about the nature of Kundalini.

At this point Western researchers readily admit that they don't know where PK comes from. Many of them openly concede that the theory of PK coming from the mind is only an *opinion* that is most likely premature. In the 1960's, Soviet scientists closely studied Nina Kulagina, a PK agent that became one of the most significant in the history of parapsychology. Scientists from the United States, Finland, and even Australia were involved in countless PK experiments with Kulagina.

Kulagina demonstrated that she could move objects across the table, displace compass needles, and make a pile of matches explode outwards by using mental efforts alone She also proved that by PK, she could separate the white of an egg, which was broken in a saline solution, from its yolk, and stop the heart of a frog from beating. The mental energy required to move objects by PK raised her pulse to 200 beats per minute, dangerously increased her blood pressure and disrupted her EEG wave pattern. These types of physical changes normally only occur when a person is under great stress. PK experiments often left Kulagina exhausted, dizzy, depressed, and harmed her eyesight. She eventually suffered a heart attack; which stopped her from participating in further experiments. I also experience great symptoms of physical and emotional stress when trying to control the refrigerator with my mind. Kulagina told Henry Gris and William Dick, the authors of The New Soviet Psychic Discoveries. "I concentrate on it. I must tune myself into the object. I feel as if some kind of energy is pouring from the sides of my fingertips, and from the sides of my hands."

She had a strong background in healing, and even claimed herself that she is a powerful healer. While she was not a medium involved with seances in particular, she was evidently spiritually awakened and quite active in metaphysics prior to the onset of her PK. According to Dr. Thelma Moss, an associate professor of psychology at the UCLA Neuropsychological Institute, Kulagina initially became aware of her PK abilities after she was involved in skin vision testing. This is a form of ESP testing that has been of long interest to Soviet scientists. It is my view based on my personal experiences with PK research that this testing somehow activated and triggered   her PK powers.

Kulagina conducted the skin vision ESP tests with Dr. L.L. Vasiliev, who was the Dean of the Soviet parapsychologists at that time. Vasiliev was a prominent parapsychologist at the Bechterev Institute for Brain Research, and also a Professor at Leningrad University. Kulagina was one of his first subjects in these experiments. Dr. Vasiliev made very notable contributions within the realm of parapsychology. He strongly encouraged Kulagina as her "Guru:" to develop her PK further. He made critical suggestions that helped her further understand her innate telekinetic powers..

Dr. Vasiliev suggested that Kulagina enhance her PK abilities by practice in deflecting compass needles. Interestingly, she was able to complete this task with ease. In fact, it became her main warm-up exercise and one of her main displays. Prior to demonstrating other powerful PK abilities, Kulagina uses this compass exercise as a warm up. During their PK studies, Kulagina noticed that she had the ability to move certain objects involved with the experiments. After discovering that she had these paranormal powers, she graduated and began applying her PK to move other small objects such as matches, vials, and many small stationary items. Before his death in the 1960's, he made many crucial contributions to the world of parapsychology. His most notable contribution was the discovery of Kulagina during his psi research.

Dr. Zdenek Rejdak, a Czech scientist from the Prague Military Institute visited Kulagina to test her PK and recorded the effects in a film. She was thoroughly searched for magnets and other foreign instruments that she could use to fake the PK. During these experiments, Dr. Rejdak reported that Kulagina made a compass needle move more than ten times, by merely holding her hands 5-10 cm above it. She then made the entire compass rotate on the table and also dislocated a matchbox, some individual matches, and a group of 20 matches simultaneously.

Dr. Rejdak further reported that he placed a gold ring on the table from his own finger. Kulagina hovered her hands above it, and she made it move faster than any of the other objects in the experiment. She also moved glass objects and other random items selected by Dr. Rejdak that were placed on a seat or the floor in full light. According to Dr. Rejdak, "threads or other attachments were out of the question... Fraud was impossible, as she was sitting in a fully illuminated room controlled by Dr. Zvenev, Mr. Blazek, and myself." Based in his experiences with Kulagina, Dr. Rejdak organized a conference on parapsychology in Prague in September 1968.

Her abilities also included: Movements of small objects, and alteration of existing motions, physiological effects, and exposure effects on photographic film. She is also able to exert telekinesis on stationary objects, levitate objects, deflect compass needles, impress letters or numerals onto photographic prints, and PK on living organisms. For example, Kulagina has been known to speed up the heart beat of a frog during PK testing. Until the 1960's, Kulagina was virtually unknown in the West.

After certain films were smuggled out of Russia and somehow came to America, US scientists grew very interested in studying her first hand. In the 1960's, Western scientists became most interested in studying Kulagina, after her films appeared across Europe. When these films were smuggled out of the Soviet Union, they first appeared in England and came to the attention of a physicist, Mr. Benson Herbert, who directed the Paraphysical Laboratory based in Dowton, Wiltshire. Herbert was the first to analyze these films in the West between 1968 and 1970. The Paraphysical Laboratory published the Journal of Paraphysics, which was the very first publication to translate Soviet scientific reports regarding parapsychology.

Scientists from around the world have witnessed Kulagina slide objects across tabletops, cause suspended ping-pong balls to gyrate behind Plexiglass tubes, produce burn marks by merely touching an observer's arm, and many other amazing feats. During these feats,

Kulagina had many physical reactions similar to the ones experienced Palladino including physical weight loss, extreme exhaustion, debilitation, convulsions and even vomiting. In 1969, Kulagina's films were presented to the Society of Psychical Research in England. Of course researchers in the Soviet Union have thoroughly studied Kulagina. The main researcher involved with her was Dr. Grenady Sergeyev of the A.A. Uktomskii Physiological Institute based in Leningrad. He theorized that PK is some kind of a biological field, and discovered that during testing Kulagina produced more electromagnetic radiation than when she is at rest. Soviet researchers have confirmed her ability to manipulate materials of any physical constitution, including metals, plastics, fabrics, and organic materials.

Soviet scientists discovered that screening or shielding objects in various ways has no effect on how Kulagina could effect them. Screening these target objects with lead-impregnated glass, paper, metal plates, wood, and other materials does not hinder her ability to affect these objects. No electrical charge has been observed around the objects that she moves with her PK. Both Soviet and Western scientists have tested Kulagina under quite controlled conditions and have confirmed all of this. Based on their full summaries of these reports, there are strong grounds for accepting her effects as valid PK.

Much support for Kulagina's claims comes from others who have succeeded in performing the same feats after observing her on film. The best example is Felice Paris, a research technician at the Maimonides Medical Center in New York who practiced at home and was eventually able to move a bottle several inches under what the researchers considered to be controlled conditions. I also have been able to move cups in my kitchen several inches by my PK. When it happens, it sort of feels like a magnet pushing another one away.

Various tests within the medical center's lab showed that Parise was one of the best ESP subjects they worked with. Following several months of persistent practice trying to move a plastic eyelash container every day, she succeeded in moving the bottle involuntarily as she reached for the container and it suddenly moved away from her hand. She later demonstrated the ability in the laboratory to rotate a compass needle using her PK. Many parapsychologists including Charles Honorton and J.G. Pratt and Mantague Ullman observed her demonstrations under informal but carefully controlled conditions.

Charles Honorton was a senior researcher at the Maimonides Lab, and he was the first to observe Parise's psychokinetic effects. She had a close bond with him based on their extensive ESP studies conducted within the laboratory. At the 1973 convention of the Parapsychological Association held in Charlottsville, Virgina, Honorton reported that he received a letter from Parise indicating her ability to displace a small alcohol bottle presumably by PK. He was invited to her home for the demonstration in New York, where she actually did move a partially filled alcohol bottle up to two inches away from her, by merely looking at it for two to three minutes.

The bottle was carefully examined to ensure that no moisture was on it causing it to glide and that nothing was attached. She repeated this feat many times during his visit. Honorton took all possible measures to ensure that trickery was not involved by examining the counter, the positioning and condition of the vial. He also reported that over the course of several months, Parise was able to replicate the feat. She also was successful in deflecting needles of small pocket compasses using her telekinetic powers. She would typically accomplish this by placing her hands cupped slightly about six inches above its surface.

Many researchers from the West began investigating Kulagina in the 1970's. Dr. J. Gaither Pratt, one of J.B. Rhine's former co-workers at the Duke University Parapsychology Laboratory was one of the first Americans to visit Paris. He was one of Rhine's closest investigators in dice throwing experiments and poltergeist cases. Although Kulagina has been available to Western researchers only sporadically and under rather informal conditions, they are confident that her PK effects are paranormal.

Ted Serios is a rather unique PK research subject from the US that was studied under very careful controls. He was a hotel elevator operator who could apparently make paranormal changes to photographic film, particularly when he is under the influence of alcohol. Interestingly enough, Kulagina was also reported to have created changes in unexposed photographic film by her PK. The paranormal effects produced by Serios have been recorded by Polaroid, television cameras, and with conventional photographic devices. The most striking effects involve cases where a picture appears on the film that corresponds to something that Serios had seen or was thinking about. During experiments, excellent controls are used to ensure that the development of the film is not done fraudulently. Often times, the film that Serios is trying to affect by using his PK comes out in all black and white, even though it seems technically impossible under the conditions that it was developed.

In this chapter we have observed how over the past one hundred years PK research has compelled the attention of some of the world's brightest scientists. Ever since the first seance studies in Victorian Times, there has not been a dull moment in this field of psi research. There are countless other examples of PK Agents that have been studied under close scientific scrutiny. However, I provide only those accounts that simply prove to readers: 1) That PK has been thoroughly researched by top scientists and 2) That it has been concluded in these studies that PK is an unquestionably real force that can actually be measured and 3) That PK is a semi physical force which comes from within the body and is controlled by the mind, and 4) That it is influenced by our thoughts to act on matter and control reality quite effectively.

I have personally witness levitation that was certainly a result of true PK. Ramana is a famous magician from Holland that I randomly encountered while riding on a tram in Amsterdam. This was the only time that I have ever seen anybody levitate in person. In fact most people have only heard of levitation but do not have the karma which allows for them to personally witness it. That is why most readers are not sure if it is real or not. I was in the same boat until I actually saw it for myself. Since I had never seen levitation in person prior to this incident, I was naturally somewhat skeptical. It is natural for us to be skeptical about things like this, but ultimately we should earnestly wish to know if it is true or not.

We have seen the pictures and read about it in fairy tales and occult pop fiction stories, but what is the honest truth about levitation? I hope that my real-life experiences provided to you on this manuscript will clarify these matters for readers, which empowers them to proceed to a higher level of metaphysical understanding. On the morning of this levitation incident, I was working very intensively with telekinetic triggers and amplifiers, by incessant chanting and other karma yoga practices. Prior to this day, I rarely ever meditated that hard or worked with that degree of intensity. Evidently, I just might have produced a powerful psychokinetic chain reaction.

Shortly after I finished chanting that same day during the afternoon, I was riding on the tram and I noticed that at least five people sitting around me were losing unconsciousness and falling asleep. I could not help but to wonder if just maybe this had something to do with me, because so many people were going to sleep at the same time all around me. Of course, they might have all been coming back from the coffee shops and "relaxed" out of their minds, but I doubt that was the case. When the tram stopped momentarily, I looked out of the window. Sure enough, I saw a yogi floating higher than six feet in the air before some people with his legs crossed. Of course, everybody who saw him looked up at him in utter amazement. I had never seen anything like this in my entire life and I immediately chalked it up to a miracle that was psychokinetically produced my intense yoga work that same morning. I had not ever chanted that intensively before on my japa mala, and suddenly this levitation phenomenon happened as soon as I did.

As the tram stopped there momentarily, I had the rarest chance to observe this feat, and to record his website address which is www.ramana.nl. He has been featured in mainstream Indian and Dutch media for his mystical powers. He is able to float objects, levitate people without making any contact with them, and produce miracles that researchers and observers can not understand or explain.

Another classic example of an yogi who has demonstrated true PK is an Indian saint named Swami Rama, who was studied by a physicist from the Menninger Foundation. Swami Rama claimed that his Master in India could, use mental effort alone to make an object move towards him or away. However he himself was only able to make the objects move in one direction or the other. When visited by the physicist, he prepared himself by fasting, "purifying" himself, and other transcendental yoga practices. This confirms how these yogic processes definitely function as the most powerful triggers of our mind over matter abilities, by activating the divine kundalini energy. In striving to master the science of mind over matter and true psychokinessis , this is useful information to have.

Similarly, I have found that the most amazing mind over matter effects occur most frequently during or shortly after my intensive yoga practice. Witnessing the levitation with Ramana is only one example of this. Another classic example is the increased frequency of the car light phenomenon and the FP, as a result of my intense yogic practice and Guru-Disciple interactions. The object to be manipulated by Swami Rama in the experiment was constructed by the physicist himself. It was a knitting needle mounted on a pivot with a strong spring. On experiment day, the scientists assembled to witness his abilities. He sat in the Lotus Position several feet away from the object. Then he gave a mantric command three times. The second time, he said the incantation, the needle on the device rotated towards him roughly ten degrees. This is very analogous to how I am able to trigger the FP to happen and cause lights to flicker by merely uttering a divine name, such as Vishnu! Of course the difference between our PK talents is that I certainly have an affinity for primarily affecting technologies such as refrigerators, lights, computers and automobiles. These sacred incantations serve as trigger of PK.

Satya Sai Baba is a great spiritual leader and widely recognized as an avatar who is well known for his telekinetic abilities. In one case a reporter in an article on thoughtaugraphy explains how his nephew once attempted to take a picture of Sai Baba. Sai Baba then predicted to his nephew that his image would not appear on the developed film plates. The reporter analyzed his nephew's film plates and confirmed that they could not be developed just as Sai Baba predicted. Many of his disciples have reported numerous inexplicable PK phenomenon connected with him and miracles of all varieties.

His aura was analyzed closely by a Kirlian photographer, and it was determined that it has properties that are most unique and supernatural. On one occasion I was blessed to have a miracle happen in connection with using Sai Baba Nag Champa soap! I showered for quite a long time with this bar of soap for the very first time. When I got out of the shower, I looked at the clock and the time was exactly 9:11 a.m. I thought it was an interesting "coincidence," and no less than a few seconds later, my refrigerator turned on and the light in my living room blacked out for a few seconds.

Paramahansa Yogananda provides excellent examples of yogic saints who displayed quite amazing telekinetic abilities in his book The Autobiography of a Yogi. One such example is an adept named Nagendra Nath Bhaduri, "The Levitating Saint." His disciples reported that before meals he would often hold the food in hand as he blessed it. He would then rise to the sealing where he floated for a while as he blessed the food.. Another example of a powerful telekinetic provided by Yogananda is Swami Pranabananda, "The Saint With Two Bodies," who displayed stunning bi-location powers. I think that The Autobiography of a Yogi is another great tool for learning about the realities of PK activity within the context of transcendental yoga, metaphysics and religion.

Chapter 5: Modern Institutional PK Research Findings

In terms of scientific experimentation, the London based Society for Psychical Research (SPR) was established in 1882. The main purpose of this organization was to formally investigate reported cases of psi phenomenon and paranormal activity. Many prominent and well-respected scientists from all over the world were compelled to join the Society including Sir William Barret, Frederick W.H. Myers, Eleanor and Henry Sidwick, and Edmond Gurney. Similar organizations have been established around the world, such as the American Society of Psychical Research.

It is well known in academe the first institutional attempts to prove PK mind over matter were conducted in 1934 by J.B. Rhine. He was an American parapsychologist from Duke University in Durham, North Carolina. Rhine launched systematic laboratory research in the field of PK, beginning with dice throwing experiments. All of his studies related to changes of objects in motion such as cards and dice.

After both Rhine and his wife earned their Ph.d's, they began working with William McDougal from England, who was the main pioneer in modern institutional PK research. Prior to Mcdougal's involvement and impact on the field, scientists generally ignored PK phenomenon. After the Rhines began working with McDougal, he was convinced that the issues related to PK research were so critical that they needed to be studied by universities all over the world, and particularly within psychology departments.

Rhine became interested in studying PK within the lab, after he was approached by a student gambler. This student claimed that he had the ability influence the outcome of the dice throw by his will power alone. In fact, the student gambler said he certainly could get the dice face to land as he wished. This one casual visit from the student directed Rhine into a whole new realm of scientific investigation in mind over matter.

In 1943, the Rhines published their first research study that introduced the term "psychokinesis" and presented affirmative findings. Many other reports on the subject quickly followed. The results compelled many researchers to follow this method and also to refine Rhine's basic approach. By the end of 1950, a host of parapsychologists and scientists from all over the globe reported data consistent with Rhine's affirmative findings for the existence of PK. Following Rhine's lead, thousands of valuable scientific studies on PK were published by both professional and private researchers

After Rhine published a monograph on ESP, which was reported by the New York Times, his relationship with Duke University was significantly affected. He eventually had to leave the Duke psychology department due to the controversial and unorthodox research that he was engaged in. Fortunately, the university made a special arrangement, where he was given a separate parapsychology division to proceed with PK and ESP research. Of course, Rhine's methods of dice throwing by hand were heavily challenged by many critics. So, he designed another experimental approach involving a more advanced method, in order to prevent what skeptics and critics called "skilled throwing" or sleight of hand.

Rhine was long fascinated with the idea of mind over matter, but he was unsure about how it could be tested. Initially, he had subjects using dice cups attempting to influence the outcome of throws. He did not select subjects that were particularly endowed with psychic abilities. Instead, subjects from the general population were tested for their mind over matter skills. Rhine eventually created the "dice-machine," which was designed to more carefully test the influence of the throwing efforts. This contraption totally eliminated all contact that subjects had with the dice. It was made of a long electrically-driven rectangular cage mounted on an axis through the middle, so that it could be rotated. Dice were loaded in the top of the machine at the beginning of experiments. When the cage rotated, the dice were thrown from one end of the cage to the other. The interior was designed so that the dice bounced around actively as they fell, to create the most random result possible.

When using the dice-throwing machine as opposed to the hand or a cup, Rhine noticed again that the PK effects were much stronger. This supports my theory that PK has a strong propensity for manifesting through technologies. In our day and age, we can expect this energy to work in marvelous ways through our increasingly advanced technologies. These new manifestations lead us to a greater understanding of this energy's true nature, and how to control it.

Rhine's main objective in these experiments was to prove that PK was real and to provide definitive proof of it. To establish this scientific basis for the existence of PK, he performed thousands of trials before he ever dared publish. Rhine developed the first scientific and systematic approach for studying PK. He was originally trained as a Botanist and decided to use his scientific background training to investigate telepathy and "ESP," which is a term that he coined in addition to psychokinesis. Incidentally, PK has been extensively tested within the field of Botany and horticulture by many scientists, such as Dr. Bernard Grad from McGill University in Montreal Canada. Many experiments in this area indicate that plants respond to thoughts. This subject is discussed further in chapter six.

In the publication of his experiments, Rhine reported that PK does not seem connected with any physical process of the brain, nor is it subject to any of the mechanical laws of physics. The results of these PK studies cannot be explained by the laws of physics because they are "transcendental" to those laws. Hence, PK is regarded by many as a nonphysical force of the mind that can act on matter in many measurable ways. Rhine surmised after many trials that PK and ESP have a lot in common and that they are not mutually exclusive. They both act independently of space, time and can control them. He discovered that ESP played a central role in the PK process, and that one signifies the presence the other.

As Rhine continued with his experiments, they consistently provided evidence in support of PK. While he did not understand the nature and properties of what was causing PK, two years of research made fully him confident of its existence. I myself have also been studying PK and the FP closely and experimentally for nearly three years by now. It also has taken me all of this time using experimental and empirical evidence to concur with Rhine that the existence of PK and mind over matter is a matter of fact. On the basis of my discoveries, I would go so far as to say that anybody who disregards the reality of PK in light of the overwhelming evidence proving it is lost in delusion. Rhine published his research studies and findings in the Journal of Parapsychology.

Although Rhines's methodology was typically informal, and many of his experiments could not be replicated, he compelled lots of positive responses from scholars around the world. Eventually, it was generally accepted within the scientific and academic communities that his studies provided conclusive evidence for the existence of PK. The prevailing trend in psi research and especially the area of PK is the use of electrical instrumentation, due to the flexibility and precision. PK placement tests were the main refinement of Rhine's original approach. Instead of monitoring if one's PK could influence the outcome of a dice throw, placement tests consider whether this force can cause the dice to fall in certain directions on a platform where they fall. Both of these approaches relate specifically to influencing objects in motion.

Between 1959 and 1976 experimentation persisted in the realm of trying to influence the falling of objects with PK. Many researchers have reported using various mechanical and electro mechanical devices for their experiments. The first systematic analysis in placement PK was conducted in 1946 by W.E. Cox, a scientist within the Institute for Parapsychology in Duramn North Carolina. He worked closely with J.B. Rhine and is notorious for constructing ingenious PK-testing apparatus and devices for parapsychological research.

Cox brings a level of ingenuity to the field of PK research that is uniquely versatile. He has developed some of the most innovative devices ever used within his experiments. For example, he reports the use of devices that record PK influences on electrical relays and electrolyte cells. He has constructed innovative PK testing devices out of car radiators, aquarium parts, straws, and type writers. He has used marbles, steel balls, dice, coins, soap film, air bubbles, and electrical systems for his PK experiments. In one report, he invented a bubble-producer, where the subjects willed for their PK to make the bubbles drift to on side or the other.

In another case, Cox invented a contraption for testing subtle micro-PK influences. He used an ordinary bathroom spray bottle that shot water through a grid structure. These grids were somehow connected to two glass tubes. Normally, these tubes would fill up with at the same rate, when the water was sprayed through the grids. In this study, Cox wanted to determine whether micro-PK influences could cause one of the tubes to fill up faster than the other. Initially, his subjects were successful at deflecting the water drops into the target tube approximately 54 percent of the time After he completed so many of these trials, it became evident that the results were statistically far greater than chance expectation could ever account for.

The very first apparatus created by Cox for PK testing was a typewriter case placed upside down. The bottom was marked off by a checker board design of numbered squares from 1 to 6. No square had the same number. In a given trial or experiment, 24 dice were tumbles from a cup in a box that released it onto the numbered platform. Subjects willed them to land on certain boxes with designated numbers. For example, a subject throwing for 3's would try to make more dice land in the box numbered 3 by willing for their PK to produce that result. Interestingly enough, Cox 's experiments were successful and subjects consistently succeeded at this task.

Another series of machines invented by Cox consisted of pendulums whose swings were mechanically timed. A slow swing would propel the counter for a longer time than would a quick one. The subjects directed their attention towards controlling the counter rather then the pendulum that controlled it. In each trial, the subjects aimed both to slow the counter down and to speed it up. At different times in the experiment, the subjects had to either slow the counter down or accelerate it. Once again Cox found that subjects succeeded at this task by using PK. He also conducted PK experiments involving a photocell or a magnetic switch that was used to measure a pendulum stroke.

Cox once invented a three tiered platform mechanism for testing PK. Dice were placed on a chute that lead to the top tier. When released they would move through the chute to the first tier, then fall down a runway to the second tier and finally land on the bottom platform. This platform was checkerboarded with all squares marked either A or B. The subjects tried to make the dice land on certain squares more often then chance could account for. Several of the dice would remain trapped in the upper tiers of the contraption, while others would make it through to the bottom.

Cox theorized that if several dice were released simultaneously, only certain ones would be significantly affected by PK. The ones that made it to the bottom were most affected. Cox believed that by using this approach, only negatively influenced dice would remain at the top, while the ones positively inflected by PK made it to the bottom. In theory, these dice would be most responsive to the specific PK commands. Subjects in these trials succeeded in causing dice to land in designated squares far more often than "chance" could account for.

Some of the staff at Duke felt that this form of placement was unduly complex and devised another more straightforward method. They developed a contraption designed to test placement alone and in only one dimension. Dice in this contraption were mechanically released at the top of a ramp, they tumbled onto a horizontal surface, and then of course scattered and came to rest in an irregular pattern. The surface where the dice landed was divided into halves, either of which could be labeled as the placement "target" for the trial. For example, if the right dice was designated as the *target*, all dice that landed on that side were counted as "psi-hits."

A Swedish Engineer named Haakon Forwald adopted this "Duke placement technique" and made many variations to it beginning in the 1950's. In fact, his studies comprise the longest and most persistent trials of PK experiments to date. He worked primarily by himself and devoted his energy in attempting to discover consistent physical patterns and relations in the PK phenomenon. By trade, Forwald is also an inventor with hundreds of international patents under his name. He grew interested in PK after witnessing group PK involving table-tipping in seance settings. He was so fascinated with these feats that he contacted J.B. Rhine, who then convinced the Swedish inventor to focus on placement P studies.

Forwald devoted most of his efforts in discovering consistent physical relations in PK phenomenon. His work can be found in a series of reports and in a comprehensive monograph. Both Forwald and Cox experimented with objects made from different substances in placement tests. This was done to examine if PK affected each substance differently. Interestingly enough, Cox noticed higher scores while using cubes made of celluloid rather than lead. Forwald found a connection between scoring and the object's "atomic weight."

Forwald was a brilliant scientist, he and applied this ingenuity in devising experiments to test PK and prove its existence. His first test in the area involved the use of a platform that led to a tabletop via a runway. A number of dice were loaded into the top of the platform and when released down the runway, they would then bounce and land on the table surface. The table surface was divided into two halves straight down the middle.

The task for the experiment was to affect which side of the table the dice landed on by simply wishing. Forwald used his will power to make the dice land on one side of the table more often than the other. He discovered that he was able to perform this PK task successfully. Hence the old cliche, "when you wish upon a star...your dreams come true." *Wishing* upon a star triggers PK and amplifies it with specific astrological and stellar "trend energies." In a replication experiment, Forwald used dice of different weights by constructing them from wood, paper, steel aluminum and other materials. However, the composition of the dice had no bearing on his performance.

Forwald designed and conducted another experiment involving dice cubes made of different materials. As he cast the dice, he willed for his PK to influence only one type of dice. For example, if he used dice composed of wood and steel, he would will for the steel ones to be affected by PK. He found that his PK affected all of the dice equally, regardless of the composition of the cubes. After completing many other tests in PK successfully, Forwald traveled to Duke University to replicate his work before neutral observers. Under stringently controlled conditions, Forwald was consistently successful at demonstrating his PK.

On the US west coast, at Stanford University, a scientist named Gertrude R. Schmeidler conducted psi research with a psychic and purported "astral traveler" named Indigo Swann. These experiments demonstrate how PK is inherently connected to psychic abilities including astral travel. So if you have ever wanted to astral project or travel into other dimensions like Carl Castaneda and many great yogis, the key is to develop your psychokinetic skills. Of course, astral projection is only one manifestation of mind over matter abilities, which these experiments with Indigo Swann indicate.

My empirical research and PK experimentation also evidences an intrinsic connection between astral traveling (tandra) and psi phenomenon. For example, I have observed that when ever I chant

Vedic mantras incessantly just before bedtime, I nearly always astral project during that night. On the other hand, we have to remember that my whole breakthrough in PK known as the FP is also a direct result of the same "mantra yoga" practices. This shows how astral projection itself is triggered by PK in much of the same way as other mind over matter phenomenon.

One group of experiments were designed to test Swann's ability to modify the temperature registered by an electric sensor (thermistor) using his PK. Three thermistors were situated in various locations in the experimental room and connected to a chart recorder. One of them was designated as the "target" thermistor. Swann was instructed on each trial to influence the target thermistors by making them either hotter or colder. Successfully affecting these would be considered "psi hits" in the experiments.

Highly significant results were achieved among the target group thermistors in these experiments. The experimenters used the most sensitive thermometers and a polygraph devices for recording temperature changes. Swann was apparently able to consistently and dramatically change the temperature even when the target thermostats were sealed in vacuum bottles, and placed more than 20 feet away from him. In these trials, he proved to several scientists that he can mentally create temperature changes in vacuum sealed thermostats.

Swann was also studied closely at Stanford Research International (SRI) in Menlo Park, to demonstrate his PK abilities to Harold Puthoff, a physicist and parapsychologist. That experiment involved a highly sensitive magnetometer buried underground within a "superconducting field" that was immune to all normal external disturbances. It was constructed with an electric coil that surrounded the core of the machine to block outside influence. It also was encased in an eight ton iron vault, set in concrete under the laboratory.

According to reports, the magnometer device was extremely well shielded, and it was unable to be penetrated by even the smallest unit of matter. The machine was designed for measuring the periodic curve of the decay of magnetic fields. Swann's initial task was to find out for himself where the apparatus was by using his ESP. He gave a description of it, which the physicists that were present accepted as accurate. Moreover, at the same time that he reported finding the apparatus, the previously regular decay curve flattened out completely.

His next task was to psychically influence the magnetic field within the device. The device contained four separate shields to block any outside influence from affecting its magnetic frequency. Signals from within the machine's magnetic field were then transferred to a chart monitor. When Swann tried to telekinetically penetrate the inside of the machine and disrupt it, the normally stable chart record showed strong fluctuations. The person who designed the machine to be totally impervious to outside influence was initially skeptical when Swann affected the magnetometer's wavelengths so radically. This designer was so shocked that he even suggested something might be wrong with the machine. He agreed to finally believe in Swann's telekinetic powers, if he could totally flatten out the magnetic readings on the machine using at will.

Swann immediately complied and completely flattened out the lines on the reader, which dazzled all of the scientists present. The results of this investigation spread outside of the scientific community like wild fire. Swann was also involved with experiments on a special PK testing machine, where he attempted to alter the generation of "electronic noise" within its circuit. Interestingly, results were not significant when he was in the same room, but improved drastically when he was moved into another room. These research findings with Swann opened many doors in research opportunities for him, including some experiments with the US government. They were interested in potential military applications of PK energy, particularly for remote viewing purposes.

Uri Geller from Israel is currently the most notorious PK practitioners and has also been involved with research at SRI. He has been involved in more controlled PK experiments involving electronic monitoring equipment than anyone else in the world. Cox and many other researchers have observed Geller bend keys and other metal objects under conditions that were considered reliable. Cox reported that he laid a key on a table and saw that it was straight, then he held it lightly with his forefinger while Geller stroked the narrower part. Cox said that "the key began to bend slowly at a point just beyond my finger, stopping above 6 degrees. Any pressure he [Geller] might have applied would have been against the direction of the bend."

A physicist named Wilburt Franklin used a scanning electron microscope to analyze the metallic composition of a platinum ring that suddenly cracked in Geller's presence. He reported that several different microscopic structures, similar to those created by very low temperatures and melting at very high temperatures all in close proximity to the fractured area. Geller was also successful at starting a watch that Cox somehow stopped by using a piece of foil. Other researchers witnessed Geller's telekinetic ability to deflect a magnometer, when his hands were merely brought near its measuring probe.

Geller had his first PK experience at the age of 3. While sitting with his mother a spoon in his hand suddenly bent and broke. He became most popular in the 1970's, and was the ideal subject for parapsychologists. He toured the world appearing on television performing several feats on stage before large audiences. After being discharged from the Israeli military, he became a youth camp counselor and impressed the children with his talents. These demonstrations led Geller to performing in schools which opened the door for other performance opportunities and made him a celebrity.

It has been reported by many people around the world that while watching Geller on television similar phenomenon are observed in objects near them. Based on the circumstances, many of these people believe that they themselves have manifested the physical changes. Many researchers have followed up on these claims and investigated them scientifically. While some of these claims were invalid, others were actually confirmed by scientists.

A special case of interest involves a young boy's ability to deform spoons that investigators placed in a sealed container. This is a feat that Geller himself seems unwilling to try. The young boy's psychic power is certainly an example of true PK. Many other researchers have also reported similar changes under very well controlled conditions. For example, researches found that the former poltergeist research subject, Matthew Manning was able to create similar metal bending effects.

Geller is also religious and he believes that his powers are a gift from God. He developed an interest for using his gift to help science, so he began submitting to numerous research studies. In 1971, he met with Andrija Puharich, a prominent American neurologist and well respected investigator of paranormal matters. He ran several tests on Geller and was firmly convinced that his powers were genuine. He then arranged to have Geller further examined at the Stanford Research Institute (SRI International) in Menlo Park to assess his psi skills. While studied at Stanford, he impressed a number of professional researchers by bending spoons, teleporting and deforming certain objects.

Geller was further examined by two more SRI researchers for telepathy, clairvoyance, and potential applications in information transmission. He was quite successful in all of this psi research. Despite the claims of many researchers in Great Britain who criticized these experiments on grounds of methodology, it was acknowledged by most that he was able to produce effects that were highly implausible. Although Geller has been accused of fraud by many, he was more formally investigated by a government researcher at the Naval Surface Weapons Center for his psychic abilities. Again, in these tests for his telekinetic powers were confirmed.

Another prominent scientists who researched Geller was John Hasted, a physics professor and head of the physics department at the University of London. He personally attested to Geller's psychic powers under highly controlled experimental conditions. An investigation team witnessed Geller effect a Geiger counter device, by sending it into convulsions with readings 500 times the normal rate by merely holding it in his hand. This was a clear indication to the scientists that the mind does influence activity on the sub-atomic "quantum" level. The research team concluded that Geller performed better in PK testing when the trials were challenging for him. They also found that the rigidity of the methodology used actually hindered him from demonstrating the fullest extent of his PK. That was only a result of his karma because in some cases as we have seen, the rigidity of the methodology has no bearing on the subject's performance.

Of course, Geller has many critics who believe that he uses sleight of hand techniques. For example, James Randi actually was able to reproduce all of Geller's abilities using certain techniques. He even wrote a book entitled The Truth About Uri Geller, which discusses how Geller could be using stage magic techniques to produce these effects. In the case of the FP discussed in this handbook, there is no possibility of any stage trickery.

No physical contact with the refrigerator is necessary for it to be effected by the PK energy. Nothing is done on stage and there are many witnesses to the feat. Hence, the FP by its nature is unequivocally a case of true PK. Moreover, the FP is far more consistent, reliable, and less evasive for monitoring, research and analysis purposes. For PK scientists this manifestation represents a whole new concept in research and potential for observation. It is directly analogous to the young boy who is able to bend the spoons at a distance.

One of the most notable advancements in PK research emerged with the advent of the Random Number Generator (RNG) built by Helmut Schmidt. He is an industrial physicist from Germany, who worked within the Boeing Institute in Seattle as a senior scientist. He then served as the director of research at FRNM, and more recently as a researcher for the Mind Science Foundation in San Antonio, Texas. Schmidt eventually adapted the original RNG invention, where electrons emitted by strontium-90 decay trigger a switch.

The main modification of this new RNG was that a two-position switch was used. Careful pretesting indicated that under controlled conditions, the two positions had random outputs. These RNG devices monitor and record PK phenomenon reflected by the discharge of radioactive particles. The RNG greatly simplifies the PK experimenter's role by presenting subjects with an interesting task, and providing quick feedback of results. It facilitates gathering a large amount of data, and provides automatic recording. The availability of the RNG stimulated and generated lots of research. Schmidt's theory about how PK effects radioactive emissions on the quantum plane has compelled attention from scientists worldwide.

RNG machines are now used to study many forms of ESP and PK. They are composed of a square-wave oscillator that stops when atomic disintegration is detected. At any random time, when atomic disintegration activates the machine, the oscillator is triggered to stop and its polarity is tested. These micro dynamic machines have continually been developed ever since Schmidt invented the first one.

Machines based on the same functioning principle used with the RNG are now being used by psi researchers around the world. In fact, at each Parapsychological Association convention, several reports are read involving research using these machines. This is all information that the general public has no knowledge of whatsoever, yet they are so quick to pass their ignorant, delusional, psychotic and uneducated judgement on matters such as PK. I encourage you not to fall pray to the devil trap of ignorance and its bi products resulting from the energies of maya that are so concentrate in this age of Kali.

These machines with only a fifty-fifty chance of success, are known as "electronic coin flippers" because the plus and minus positions could also be regarded as heads or tails and sometimes register in this way. That configuration makes more sense to subjects and causes them to feel more comfortable using the machine. Prior experience with PK is not necessary for effectively using RNG devices. For example, in 1976 Scott Hill from the University of Copenhagen in Utrecht reported a case involving a teenage girl with no prior record or experiences with psi. Within two days, she completed over 13,600 trials with the RNG and scored 172 times above what the element of chance could statistically account for.

In 1977, 18 papers were read at the Parapsychology Convention in Washington D.C. Out of these eight reports, ten of them concerned PK research. Eight of the ten PK reports involved the use of micro dynamic RNG machines. In 1975, Charles Honorton summarized sixteen PK studies where Schmidt-type machines were employed. The studies were conducted between 1970 and 1975. In thirteen of the experiments, over eighty percent gave extremely significant results. In these studies, there was less than one chance in ten billion that the results could have been achieved by chance.

More recently, machines have been developed that can distantly measure tension, which is reflected by galvanic skin response (GSR) and muscles tension (EMG). Brain waves are reflected on machines by EEG's, and many other physiological processes. These recordings are commonly charted alongside a PK results graph. This makes it simple to see whether any particular physiological traits are associated with PK. This kind of equipment has been used in research conducted at laboratories around the world, such as the Psychophysical Research Laboratory (PRL) at Princeton Forrestal Center, in New Jersey.

Schmidt's research marked the beginning of a new direction in parapsychology, which involved the study of subatomic particles. He was privileged to work closely in the field with J.B. Rhine at Duke. Parapsychologists prior to Schmidt failed to demonstrate that a known physical force was responsible for PK. Some researchers suspected that the force might be related to gravity. Parapsychologists eventually classified PK and ESP as large scale "quantum events" within the field of physics.

His findings eliminated some of the ambiguity that confused earlier investigators in the field of PK. Over time, many scientists hypothesized that the more random and unpredictable the movement or process, the stronger the PK effect would be. Although there has been over a century of research in the West conducted in the field of PK, no parapsychologist has yet adequately explained how the mind interfaces with the forces that literally shape the revelry of reality. On the other hand once again, the world scriptures of the Vedanta are a rich source of this transcendental knowledge. It is a challenging task for modern researches to account for what forces could be causing the strange phenomenon related to PK.

By analogy, many researchers suggest that in the world of sub-atomic particles, things are also unpredictable and no less bizarre than teleportation or levitation on the physical level. We have seen how some researchers have demonstrated how people claiming to be gifted psychics can objectively effect the behavior of these particles on a subatomic level. Researchers hypothesize that if these powers manifest on the subatomic levels that control matter, this effect might carry over to the physical plane as well. This analogy seems interesting, but modern researchers claim that the laws of the subatomic world can not directly be applied to the larger macro-world.

As I became more intrigued by the connections between science, technology and spirituality, I considered conducting a psychotronics experiment while living in Amsterdam, Holland. I intended to project the subtle energies from a mantra given by my Dutch Guru onto my own energetic/pranic body. This heavy duty machine also enables the user to change brainwaves using frequency technologies, so I used it to induce an altered state while projecting the mantric energy. I knew that this mantra was all powerful, so I hesitated before conducting this experiment for several weeks based on fear of the unknown. I grew unbearably curious about the metaphysical effects of such an experiment. So, one random day, I felt more daring than ever! I actually performed this psychotronic test using this Hare Krsna Vedic mantra. That very same random day that I finally conducted this experiment, I was riding my bicycle through the city, and I heard loud drumming and singing.

I liked the sound of the music and decided to follow the vibration. As I approached this rare event, I realized that it was an enormous and very rare Hare Krishna festival that attracted "devotees" from all over the world. There was a very large crowd of people from all over the world right in the heart of Amsterdam celebrating Lord Sri Krsna, the very same day that I did my experiment using the Hare Krishna Maha Mantra. At that point, I realized that the mantra was very powerful, that the technologies are quite real, and that they obviously can influence material things including events. This is a great example of how the mind can directly influence matter under certain times and conditions.

Currently, one of the most active sections of psi research is its study of altered states of consciousness. Interestingly enough, in the larger field of psychology as a whole, there is proportional level of interest proliferating in studying altered states. After reviewing literature on psychical research, many scientists are amazed at the strong connections between altered states if consciousness and psi phenomenon. Many scientists theorize that certain altered states of consciousness are conducive to response factors in the mind that heighten or trigger psi effects. In fact, L.E. Rhine has conducted thousands of spontaneous studies of ESP that evidence how more of it occurs in altered states of consciousness such as dreams, as opposed to the normal waking state. These studies involved variables such as certain stimulation to reduce attentiveness for external distraction, reduction of internal distractions through relaxation and meditation techniques, and the redirecting of one's focus internally.

Many parapsychologists have even attempted to enhance ESP scoring by studying subjects in altered states of consciousness such as those in the sleeping state, those who have been drugged, placed in sensory bombardment or sensory deprivation environments, or subjects undergoing biofeedback training or meditation. Even in the wider world of psychology, there is an unprecedented increased in altered states. Modern parapsychologists have determined in research studies that certain brainwave activity is more closely associated with PK, enhanced mind power, and many other psychic manifestations. Naturally, people have taken advantage of this specialized knowledge by learning how to alter brain waves for certain purposes.

This relationship between mind and matter is fascinating and exciting. It can be quite useful when we consider that there are now a wide range of technologies available which are specifically designed to control the brain waves. Shakti Yoga is a matter of understanding how the divine energy functions on all levels in relation to the mind. As a human being it is your spiritual duty to optimize the use of your internal technologies to make the world a better place and your life as blissful as possible. Fortunately, there are now technologies that are specifically designed to immediately alter brain waves using life energy apparatus and frequency based technologies. These can be powerful tools for enabling us to control the mind's frequency at will for whatever purpose needed.

While only a few studies done have analyzed the effects of drugs on psi performance, considerable work has been done involving hypnosis. Most of these studies conducted have found that the hypnotic state is closely associated with ESP scoring. Other studies have found additional connections between ESP, hypnotic susceptibility and the depth of the hypnotic experience. This explains why druids, shamans and conjurors induce altered states through drumming and other rituals before phenomenal spiritual powers are unleashed.

When we take this to a more advanced technological level, away from the realm of the indigenous world, we can wield even more control over these supernatural God given mind powers using modern technology. I openly encourage my disciples and readers to safely experiment and run tests in altering your brain waves for spiritual advancement and greater control over material nature (maya). The four major types of brain waves are Beta, Alpha, Theta, and Delta which are all described below.

Beta (i.e. 13.1 Hz): Characterized by brain waves that are shorter and have closer peaks. When one is often awake and alert such as walking, talking, dancing, or during periods of acute anxiety or stress the brain usually stays in this mode. Can be used to foster efficiency and high energy levels.

Alpha (i.e. 7.83 Hz or 7.0 Hz): These brain waves are most closely associated with PK phenomenon. This state is induced by hypnosis, meditation, listening to music or watching television. Also, associated with ESP and superior creative abilities.

Theta (i.e. 3.5 Hz or 6.3 Hz): Associated with deep trance, which some mystics can induce at will. Pain is dulled when theta waves predominate. That is why many mystics can endure great pain after inducing this mind state (i.e. walking on coals or sitting on nails.) Theta is also associated with superior learning.

Delta (i.e. 2.5 Hz or 3.0 Hz): Slower than the other brain wave states and usually generated during sleep. When the brain is endangered by injury or disease, it may lapse into delta-wave state

Since the 1930s, interest in PK has increased and created the most active area of research in parapsychology. This is particularly true within the Soviet Union and the United States. It is also being researched heavily by biologists, physicists, engineers, and the phological community, along with many private researchers. It has become apparent to many that if PK force is brought under sufficient control it has potentially unlimited applications.

All over the planet we see examples where physics, science and related technology is being used to investigate psychic activity. Of course, technology is not merely used in the research, observation, and discovery phase involved with any energy or natural resource. It is obviously needed for the exploitation and utilization of these power sources. As a result, science is constantly considering how modern technological capabilities can be used to generate, control, amplify and maximize PK force and its potential.

By now, the direction of formal PK research is heading in one main direction; the development of technologies called "psychotronics," where a known form of energy (i.e. prana or electromagnetic energy) is used to amplify a person's PK, who otherwise would have low to average PK levels. This gives these people far greater psychic and supernatural abilities. The term psychotronics in this context implies a marriage between the latest breakthroughs in the field of psi and the most advanced modern engineering capabilities. The "psycho" aspect of the term denotes subtle energies that are controlled and produced by the mind. The "tronics" aspect of this term refers to technologies and engineering capabilities.

Actually, psychotronics literally refers to the study of subtle energy fields, waves, forces, and frequencies, such as PK that are emitted from the human brain. Psychotronic apparatus are very powerful devices that can instantly amplify and control these energies if used properly. This empowers one to control matter more easily, significantly influence events at any distance, and experience a wide range of other psi phenomenon. This is all discussed extensively in the final chapter of this book.

Telekinetic energy has been studied by many researchers and cultures around the world under various labels. For example, Franz Anton Mesmer called it with "animal magnetism," Karl von Reichenbach named it "Od" or "Odyl," and Dr. Wilhelm Reich found it was labeled it as "orgone energy." In all three cases, they are referring to the very same energy, prana that triggers the awakening of divine Kundalini energy. This energy has been analyzed and mastered by yogic adepts, sages, gurus and masters for centuries. That is why the psychical and physical manifestations of this same life force are nearly identical to mind over matter phenomenon associated with prana. Most people don't know that when they practice yoga, they are automatically working with prana and strengthening their mind over matter skills.

The belief in an all pervading universal force became popular in European thinking in the eighteenth century, when Mesmer discovered " Mesmerism." This term refers to a psycho-physiological state which is regarded as hypnosis today. Mesmer used various kinds of magnets passing over subjects bodies which would induce trance. This is partially due to the funny relationship between electricity and magnetism. Remember that our brains and bodies function on small electric impulses. Electric currents make magnetic fields and shifting magnetic fields can induce currents. Many researchers have found that "electromagnetic technologies" have the potential to alter brain waves, to amplify thought power and also trigger PK. That seems to have been Mesmer's claim to fame in his healing work. These technologies can have a strong beneficial effect on the bio-energetic field and can release certain energy blockages that lead to other complications.

Many people are unaware that the basis of Mesmer's work involved complex theories about a magnetic fluid that permeated the body and the entire universe. He believed that magnets were able to act upon this fluid and that man could project it onto other people and inanimate objects. The FP is some form of evidence that the energy can definitely affect inanimate objects. In terms of modern breakthroughs in the area of magnetic energy technology, there are some phenomenal new concepts. For example, there are certain products that work with the magnetic field of the body and have been reported by users to drastically improve their overall well being and mental powers. On one occasion I was invited to a meeting where certain electromagnetic devices were on display and testimonials were given by the users. During the seminar there were reported cases of phenomenal health benefits and healing as a result of using these cutting edge technologies.

Many of these testimonies involved relief from chronic pain, muscle spasms, sleeping and eating disorders, along with many other unpleasant conditions. While the products were not purported to correct any health related issues in substitute for traditional medicine and a primary physician, people did report that they were effectively healed. On the day of the seminar, a miracle happened that I believe was directly connected to these electromagnetic breakthroughs. Several hours before the meeting, I had a discussion with the person who invited me regarding metaphysics. During our brief discussion, I just happened to mention the concept of "water-witching," which is "dowsing" for water with a rod. I explained water witching to him in relation to "pendulum dowsing."

Later on that night at the seminar, there was a rather large crowd of people. Out of nowhere, I was randomly selected to come up for a magnetic product demonstration with a man from India, who was very familiar with all of them. During his brief presentation, he had me hold the device in hand, and passed some kind of magnetic wand over me to clear out my energy field. Then out of nowhere, while he was describing the technologies, he just happened to mention water witching. I was quite surprised and immediately pointed out that earlier that same day I just started talking about water witching with the guy that invited me. The man who invited me was amazed by this thought transfer phenomenon as well. Then again, maybe it was only a "coincidence." Some people were clearly amazed at this apparent psychic experience. Although this may seem like a mere coincidence to many, I know based on my experience and expertise in telekinesis that this was a telepathic effect caused by the machines that acted as triggers for that psychic interchange.

Very significant contributions to this field of science were made by a German scientist named Karl von Reichenbach (1788-1869). He wrote may books on subjects such as magnetism and electricity, and conducted experiments with many psychically endowed individuals.

The main difference in approach between Rhine and Reichenbach was that Rhine used ordinary people, while Reichenbach used subjects that with strong psychic skills. Reichenbach followed up where Mesmer left on in his discoveries and research.

Reichenbach believed that life energy (a.k.a. prana) has the following properties: It is universal force that pervades all matter; it can not be eliminated from anything; electricity, friction and many other specific sources of power can concentrate it; It has polarity; It can radiate over any distance and conducts through metals, glass and fabric; It can be transferred from one body to another; it is often luminous and visible; it is especially harnessed within the human body. It is fascinating to note how both Mesmer and Reichenbach experienced psychic phenomenon during their investigations and experiments.

In more recent times, Dr. Wilhelm Reich a Freudian psychoanalyst, has contributed significantly to our understanding of the energies involved with PK. He sought to find tangible evidence for the existence of the very same universal force studied by Reichenbach and Mesmer. While studying human sexuality, he discovered the existence of this life energy he called orgone. He shared similar views with Reichenbach his predecessor in terms of his beliefs that this life energy pervades all space in the universe; and that it can exert physical psychokinetic effects on man, plants and inanimate objects.

While working at the University of Oslo in Norway during the 1930's Dr. Reich maintained that he discovered the basic units of life energy which he called bions. Reich's research generated considerable controversy after he constructed apparatus that accumulate this energy which he used specifically for healing patients of cancer. These accumulators were simply boxes lined with layers of organic and inorganic materials. He believed that by sitting in the box or placing a diseased limb inside of it, the energy would permeate the tissue and facilitate healing diseases such as cancer.

That was his personal health related opinion, which ultimately led to the destruction of his works and his incarceration. In many countries such as the US, it is illegal to use psychotronics for healing purposes, but in other places such as the UK and continental Europe, it is perfectly legal. Reich also developed certain energy devices to control the weather which gave rise to his cloud busting experiments. Even Albert Einstein became interested in Reich's work. Reich believed that life energy (a.k.a. prana) was a universal force that could be controlled to help benefit the planet in countless ways.

Reich's research continuous until this day at his laboratory in Maine which he founded. In recent years there has been resurgent interest in Reich's work and experiments. For example, Dr. Bernard Grad, Reich's former associate has tried to continue with the less controversial research. The next logical step after effectively accumulating prana energy with certain apparatus is the development of methods for generating it. Some scientists from Europe, and Russia in particular have invented ingenious devices for generating this life force. These psychotronic inventions have been a major part of my advancements in PK practice, Shakti yoga and in my spiritual realization. Although these powerful energetic devices can theoretically make anything happen, I espouse that the most intelligent application of this cosmic force is for spiritual advancement.

Chapter 6: PK and Healing Among Humans

Many religious scholars contend that PK is really a "spiritual gift" Various stories in the Bible confirm that PK has some intrinsic connection with spirituality. For example, the story where Paul and Silas escaped from prison and their bands were released in Acts 16. Other religions around the world have also reported cases of psychokinesis including astral projection among the shamans, levitating/flying yogis, poltergeists and various healing in churches.

Based on my personal experiences with PK and my discoveries in this field, I concur that it is a bi-product of spiritual advancement and yogic practice.

This chapter discusses the correlations between PK and faith healing. The annals of time are filled with inexplicable accounts of spontaneous and miraculous healing. These have obviously occurred under a wide array of circumstances ranging from Orthodox Christian settings to new age alterative environments. Many people for one reason or another are specifically endowed with that healing touch based on the complexities of their karma. According to the precepts of Mahayana Buddhism that we studied earlier in this handbook, this subjective aspect of the healer's karma is nondifferent from the external objective world.

Apparently there is some truth to this Buddhistic theory concerning the relationship between objective and subjective worlds. Witches have been burned alive because they displayed healing powers and the opposite effects on people. Shamans and witch doctors from indigenous cultures are still the source of healing for many who validate their powers. Faith healers in many churches circles are known for the ability to create these phenomenal effects for people in dire need.

Psychic healers, spiritual healers, faith healers, and Christian Scientists all believe that they can help people recover from sickness through some spiritual or religious process. Many people believe that they have been miraculously healed by the actions of faith healers. The main problem in the area of healing in humans is that there is a dearth of laboratory, clinical, and scientific research to substantiate it. This lack of scientific proof makes it really difficult to determine whether PK is the specific factor responsible for healing in humans.

The majority of information that we have regarding miraculous healing in humans comes from empirical research that is based on observation or "first hand experience." For example, Lourdes is a place in southwestern France where people have been healed, or thought that they have been healed by paranormal means. Every year between March to October the Sanctuary of Our Lady of Lourdes or the Domain (as it is most commonly known) is the place of mass pilgrimages from Europe and other parts of the world.

The spring water from the grotto is believed by some to possess healing powers. A common misconception is that miracles are the core of the Sanctuary of Lourdes, and the reasons for visits. Although this is probably the case for some visitors, the majority of pilgrims come as part of their Christian faith, and to help those in need. There have been from the beginning skeptics of the miracles reported to have taken place in Lourdes. The Roman Catholic Church has officially recognized 68 miraculous cases of healing at the Lourdes Shrine.

I think that the most striking empirical research record about miracles at Lourdes was the case of a Belgian man. His left leg had been broken when he fell from a tree. A compound fracture resulted, which later became infected, but he refused to allow the amputation of the leg. Although the poor man could hardly even move because of the injury, he made a pilgrimage to Lourdes in 1875. Before this journey was undertaken, a surgeon Dr. Affenaer removed a piece of fragmented bone that was trapped within the break of the leg. After the bone was removed, there was a one-inch separation between the two parts of the leg bone which caused him unbearable pain. Doctors believed that amputation was the only answer. In fact, one witness, Dr. Van Hoegstenberghe examined him in 1875 and reported:

"Rudder had an open wound at the top of the leg. In this wound one could see the two bones separated by a distance of three centimeters. There was no sign of healing. Pierre was in great pain and suffered this since eight years before. The lower part of the leg could be moved in all directions. The heel could be lifted in such a way as to fold the leg in the middle. It could be twisted, with the heel in front and the toes in back, all these movements being only retrained by the soft tissue."

This opening in de Rudder's leg was continually examined up until a week before his journey to Lourdes. Upon arriving at the shrine, de Rudder's injured leg was in the worst position ever. Its dangling had irritated the limb to no end. He finally prayed in a state of spiritual ecstacy, while walking up to the statute of the Virgin at the Lourdes facilities. Due to the nature of his injuries, his maneuvering would not have been possible under normal conditions. That was the point where he recognized that he was healed. His family was astounded, and Drs. Affenaer and Dr. Van Hoegstenberghe were dumbstruck, which is an understatement. It was medically impossible for the leg to heal, but it is was somehow healed instantly and miraculously.

Pierre died in 1898, and the next year Van Hoestenberghe was granted permission to exhume the body in order to analyze the healed leg. The doctor amputated both legs and the photographs are still available. They very clearly show that the bones in the left leg are deformed, but have been fused over by a new piece of healthy bone that somehow grew and merged the severed ones. This is remarkable because the healing was of a condition that was not curable by any ordinary means.

It is also interesting to note how some kind of psychic process must have played a part in the cure. Spontaneous recovery can not account for the regrowth of new bones. This case is also fascinating because it is apparent that some intelligent and willful force was involved that resembles PK in many ways. This force obviously knew exactly what was necessary to repair de Rudder's complex injuries. It is striking how this process is similar to the way PK works so intelligently. Physical acts and intelligent ones are also created through the agency of PK.

Aside from the de Rudder case, only a handful of cases recorded at Lourdes or anywhere else for that matter appear to be related to PK or anything paranormal. This form of healing is far less common than many religious sects would have the public believe. Most of the empirical reports from the Lourdes are provided in *Eleven Lourdes*

Miracles, by Dr. D.J. West a British psychiatrist. He argues that sloppy documentation was involved with most of the cases recorded at the Lourdes. In all of the cases, he found that the medical records for the patients were too insufficiently detailed for him to make proper outside evaluation.

In some cases, the original diagnosis were suspect. In other cases, the follow up investigations on the lasting effects of the cures were too insufficient to mean anything at all. Some of the patients were healed of disorders where spontaneous remission is fairly common. Since none of the eleven cases met his standard for evidence, West felt justified in rejecting all of them as untrustworthy accounts and his conclusions of Lourdes are almost totally negative.

Dr. D.J. West reported:

"The rarity of the cures, and the incompleteness of the medical information on most of the cases put forward as miraculous makes any kind of appraisal exceedingly difficult. As far as it goes, and taking the dosier at their face value, the evidence for anything miraculous in the popular sense of the expression is extremely meager."

These are typical difficulties confronted by any scientist who hopes to document irrefutable proof of paranormal healing. Despite his negative investigation of Lourdes, Dr. West does believe that some people have had recoveries there, but does not feel that they are in any way miraculous. As a psychiatrist, he argues that the recoveries might be telling us something very interesting about the regenerative powers of the mind and body. Lourdes of course is not the only place where people believe that they have been miraculously healed. Many people claim to have been healed by manifestations of faith healers. An ideal example of this is illustrated in a video by Louis Hay entitled *You Can Heal Your Life*. In this video, three Chinese Doctors (Healers) somehow focused their PK energies on a woman who had a malignant tumor growing within her. Apparently, this was documented on film and the tumor simply vanished in 3 minutes! Unfortunately however, most spiritual healing practitioners are unable to prove their claims when analyzed scientifically. Nor have they setup their own experiments to prove it. To further illustrate this problem, consider one report, where Dr. Louis Rose, a British physician scientifically researched the late Harry Edwards, one of England's most famous psychic healers.

The study focused on 95 patients who were treated and allegedly helped or "healed" by Edwards. Dr. Rose was not able to obtain medical records for fifty-eight of the patients. In twenty two of these cases, the claims of the patient were totally different from what their medical records indicated. Three patients improved but relapsed. In another four cases, the patients improved that were treated,. but they were also undergoing conventional medical treatment at the time same they were "touched" by Edwards. Only three patients were left whose improvement might have been due to Edward's healing. This was not enough information to determine conclusively whether anybody was cured.

Many people do not realize how sensitive to psychological factors many diseases are. Cancer is one of the most dreaded diseases of our era. However, most forms of cancer are curable by orthodox medicine and certainly can be prevented. Following the guidelines of *Bhakti-yoga* is one of the best means of warding off illnesses such as cancer and aids. By simply following the regulative principles of *Bhakti-yoga* (no meat eating, no elicit sex, no intoxication, and no gambling) as a standard for life, one avoids the greatest maladies and calamities. By now, it is common knowledge within the international medical community that meat eating does cause cancer. Of all types of meat, the cow eat is the most carcinogenic and the worst for your health and for the spirit-soul.

Dairy, nuts, lentils or beans with rice, tofu, hemp products, and a wide variety of other meat substitutes are excellent sources of protein. That is much cleaner than devouring any old piece of meat you just happen to stumble onto. Some people are under the impression that they can simply bless their food before eating it and that removes the impurities. I strongly dissent based on my knowledge of the science of God, and His specific yogic injunction for living as a vegetarian. The Lord will not bless anything such as steak or pork that He expressly disapproves of! Moreover, cancer is extremely sensitive to our psychological fluctuations. Mental states and emotions plays a powerful instrumental role in the development of cancer. So, by learning to control the mind, we can markedly reduce the chances of its development. Transcendental yoga is the key to mind control, and attenuating the self from potentially harmful emotions.

Consider the following examples related to cancer and psychology:.

-By the 1930s, many French cancer specialists concluded that cancer may be triggered by certain emotional traumas.

-During the1950's, psychologist and cancer researcher, Dr. Lawrence LeShan found widowed and divorced people had a higher probability for developing cancer that the married or single. These findings revealed to him that those who have experienced deep psychological loss are more likely to develop cancer.

-In a another study, Le Shan and Dr. R.E. Worthington discovered that 62 percent of their patients developed cancer shortly after the trauma caused by loss of a spouse or some other emotionally significant relationship.

-David Kissen, who is a prominent lung cancer specialist discovered that the majority of his cancer patients did not have adequate outlets for emotional discharge," and that played an important role in their illnesses.

Many more studies suggest that psychological trauma is somehow related to cancer. However, theses five examples support my contention that cancer is somehow linked to psychological trauma and emotional distress. This is why many people wonder whether the psychotherapy process can help to eliminate cancer. Some promising leads have already been made by Dr. Carl Simonton, while working at the Travis Air Force Base Hospital. His cancer treatment seems really simple. He instructs patients to meditate, to focus attention on the cancer while willing it to dissolve. He trains his subjects in relaxation and imagery exercises. He found that a vast majority of patients who cooperate in these exercises improve!

Some recoveries in his studies are breathtaking. On the other hand, he discovered that the uncooperative patients don't seem to benefit from the procedure at all. This indicates that attitude also plays a role in the onset of illnesses like cancer. Attitude is a reflection of our spiritual disposition; yoga and meditation are really for the purpose of spiritual purification. Based on Simpton's research, it does appear that meditation, relaxation, and spiritual cleansing including yogic practice empowers the body to combat cancer. Sometimes, Simpton's has discovered that patients have been able to reduce the size of their own cancerous tumors up to 50 percent after only one week's meditation.

So, what does all of this have to do with PK? Well, it concerns the problem we have when trying to isolate a PK variable in any single case of "psychic healing." It indicates that spiritualistic healing is a complicated psychological as well as biological process that even medical authorities do not fully understand.

It is quite clear that many factors and variables are involved with the process of miraculous healing including biological, physiological, psychophysiological, and psychological. In fact, so many variables complicate the biological healing process that it is nearly impossible to isolate what role PK has, if any, in cases of spontaneous or paranormal healing. My view on this point is that telekinetic energy has been proven by many researchers cited within this handbook to effect light energies in constant motion that are randomly generated. Human emotions certainly meet this description, as they are very randomly generated and constantly in motion. By nature emotions are "light" because they connect with our thoughts and chemical processes that are constantly in motion.

. This highlights the ways in which PK energy can directly affect the emotions which have a direct bearing on health. The best way to become transcendental to the lower emotional forces is to chant the Holy Names God incessantly. *Hare Krsna Hare Krsna Krsna Krsna Hare Hare Hare Rama Hare Rama Rama Rama Hare Hare!* That mantric sacrifice situates the mind and emotions on a transcendental platform. Lord Sri Krsna is the master of the senses and when we serve Him, then He takes care of our senses and emotional issues. In addition, there is ample evidence suggesting that chanting tends to lower the blood pressure. The chief yogic scriptures reveal that the wisest ones among us chant congregationally in the temples known as *ashrams*. It is the perfect sacrifice to God known as "japa," which He will always reciprocate you for in the form countless miracles, the greatest of fortune, and the highest degree of control over material forces of nature!

While Simonton's patients very well could be using some sort of PK on themselves, it is impossible to prove it definitively. However, I have proven that PK can be triggered by chanting and other spiritual work outlined in chapter twelve. Since it is not possible to prove scientifically, we should avoid suggesting that PK alone is responsible for healing in humans. However, as reasonably thinking people, we also should not dismiss the possibility that PK could be a central factor in the healing process. Again, I think it is very effective to use PK for emotional healing and protection, which we know will improve the health overall. In this age of Aquarius that is so dominated by the element of emotion, it is no wonder that the vast majority of deaths in the West are products of degenerative illnesses such as cancer and heart disease.

As I previously stated, everyone has unique karma that accounts for our capabilities. When one person perceives another one's karmic healing powers, which are totally unfamiliar and even terrifying, one naturally resists. The most crucial thing to remember about these feats is not to be distracted by them or deluded from the main issue. One of the main purposes of this book is to highlight that even major perpetual miracles such as the FP should not be allowed to distract our attention away from the transcendental form of God. In many Eastern parts of the world miracles are called "siddhis" and are generally known by the definition provided in the *Yoga Sutras of Patanjali.*

While these are quite dramatic events when they occur, they do little to improve the human condition and a great deal to enhance human hubris. This is why the doctrines of yoga teach that their acquisition (which may spontaneously accompany enlightenment) be followed by their dismissal. Otherwise the adept can become distracted by their own phenomenal displays and potentially lose sight in the quest for integral reality. I think that rather than dismissing them entirely, the time has come to examine the nature of siddhis in a more informed and productive way. In one study concerning the nature of miracles, twelve mediators were found to have had consistent experiences of unitize consciousness and were designated as "clear" group for experimental purposes.

This clear group reported the occurrence of siddhis as well as "witnessing sleep," a state of lucid dreaming and full conscious awareness while sleeping. They also demonstrated greatly increased fluency of creative and original thought. There was a significant correlation between high creativity and the number of expected siddhis. I consider this as proof that the energy involved with producing siddhis, which certainly includes PK Force, also works within the mind telekinetically and telepathically to bring us creative imagination from the world of ideas. Perhaps it can bring us mere thoughts that empower us to resolve miseries and heal our problems.

The main issue is that we are all a part of this illusion and can control it in our own way based on our Karma. For me, the FP is something that people are subjected to in the objective world as it is a part of the very fabric of my personal Karma. Other telekinetic feats are really no different, which is why everybody is able to witness them.

Some people can heal, others can levitate, while others can affects electronics and high tech apparatus such as refrigerator units, light bulbs, power plants and automobiles. Some feats are just more subtle and less obvious, such as the purported ability to construct technologies that actually generate life force (prana energy) to amplify PK. I can not overstate how this all is a result of individual distinct karma, which is something that can be changed, improved, and enhanced through disciplinary yogic practice. While I refuse to pass any personal judgement on another's dharma, ministry, religion or spirituality, I do think that all instances of PK should be objectively and neutrally analyzed.

When Western science initially delved into the realm of psychic and spiritualistic healing, they dismissed it as sheer nonsense. They believed that these claims of miraculous healings were a result of a patient's stroke of good luck, or the skill of spiritual adepts in alternative forms of medicine. Over time, Western science and medicine came to acknowledge that perhaps some rituals and ceremonies actually do have an effect on psychosomatic illnesses in patients; they thought maybe that this accounts for many cases of miraculous healings. In their view, there was virtually no other way for inexperienced healers to cure people.

Spiritualistic healers use various approaches for achieving success in subjects. Some prefer the direct laying on of hands, others use magnets, under the belief in an energy flow that they are able to project onto the patient. Many spiritual healers, myself included, believe that this energy is a distinct force from God that we can learn to channel, control and project at any distance. Other prayer healers believe that working on people at a distance, such as by telephone, physical mail or even Internet communication works just as well or even better than the direct physical contact.

It is well known that about 85 percent of illnesses will get better, regardless of whether they are treated by a physician or not. Many religious people are quite skeptical of the medical profession at large for one primary reason alone: God has designed the body with a phenomenal system of healing itself. With sufficient time, rest and adequate conditions, the body can handle nearly anything. We can not overlook the emotional and psychological basis of healing. Healers have immense psychological effects on people, where many of them feel as though they have been cured, even though the doctor does not recognize it. An example is when we feel that something is wrong with our health, and then visit a doctor who assures us that nothing is wrong at all. Suddenly, there is psychological and emotional relief, where the patient relaxes and immediately feels better.

Some physicians are educated about the existence of PK, and they suspect that it might have something to do with a patient's miraculous recovery. In their view, the healer simply uses his personal psychokinetic powers via the agency of will power to help sick or injured people recover. However, it is also possible for the sick or injured person to facilitate their own healing by the strength of their own will. One great example of this was a relative by marriage named who had cancer and was supposedly going to die within a short time. As she laid on her hospital bed awaiting death, she began praying and wishing intensely that God would heal her right then and there. Interestingly enough, when the doctor came back into the room, he noticed that the cancer was in remission, and she was released to go home immediately. She made a full recovery and is alive and well today.

There is similar story in my family where another relative by marriage also got cancer. She received the constant healing prayer energies from many people who prayed to God for her healing. She experienced a phenomenal and miraculous full recovery of her life threatening illness. As you can see, it is no problem for the Lord to heal sickness and for PK to work in this religious context in the most phenomenal ways. Yoga is the highest form of union with God, where certain dietary and lifestyle regulations such as strict vegetarianism make the development illnesses such as heart disease and cancer far less likely. Its practices and processes also empower the yogi to wield control over the emotions and become liberated from their potentially hazardous influences. Although these relatives were not involved with yoga, they are indeed interesting cases of mind over matter, and how it works especially well in cases of great need.

In the traditional Westernized Judeo-Christian environment, there are no disciplinary regulations concerning diet at all, which is not in line with the real principles of religion derived from the Vedanta. Do you expect me to believe that this highly undisciplined lifestyle is in accordance with God's most transcendental prescriptions for living? In Bhakti Yoga for example, the main four pillars are: No meat eating, no intoxication, no illicit sex, and no gambling. It is interesting to note how all of these have direct effects on the emotional condition. The restriction on meat eating is based on the idea that vegetarianism creates a more light vibration that is conducive to the yogic endeavors.

It is apparent how these restrictions on one's life naturally control the consumption of harmful substances into our bodies. They also help to regulate the emotional states. Lord Sri Krsna has naturally set in place a system of royal yoga that if followed correctly can lead us to perfect physical health, mental and spiritual wellness. Still if we violate His principles in extreme ways and get sick because of it, His transcendental energy is powerful enough to cure any illness. However, we should not abusively violate the regulative religious and yogic principles.

Since there are so many variables involved with cases of psychic healing, (i.e. the patient's subjective attitudes, individual body chemistry, etc.) not many studies have been conducted in the area. However, Delores Krieger, a professor of nursing from New York University conducted full scale experiments, where the hemoglobin properties of diseased subjects were analyzed before and after the laying on of hands by purported healers. Control groups of those that were not subjected to the laying on of hands also had their hemoglobin checked at comparable times for changes in value. Krieger hypothesized that the hemoglobin values would change for the group subjected to the laying on of hands, but not for the control group. It turned out that she was right. In her first two studies, the difference in before and after hemoglobin levels had a probability of one in a hundred. In her third experiment the statistical difference between the two groups was one in a thousand!

Next, Krieger became curious about weather ordinary people could produce similar results in the hemoglobin properties. So, she selected thirty-two nurses each to work with two patients. The nurses were divided into two groups. The experimental group practiced their healing touch on the two patients, while the control group did not make any attempts. At the beginning of the study, there was no statistical difference in hemoglobin values between the experimental and control groups.

The differences were measured once again before and after the application of the "therapeutic touch." The differences were so drastic that they could only happen by chance in one in a thousand cases. Comparable blood samples drawn from the control group showed no significant variation. This made it appear that the therapeutic touch actually does have some effect on hemoglobin properties.

Chapter 7: PK and Biological Research:

Krieger was inspired to begin PK research by her mentor Dr. Bernard Grad, from McGill University in Montreal. He has been deeply involved with PK research involving plants, fungus cultures, and mice. Grad conducted many of his experiments with a man named Colonel Oscar Estebany, who evidently had healing powers. Estebany discovered his karmic propensity for healing as an officer in the Hungarian calvary. He noticed that lame horses seemed to recover, after he held their injured legs in his hands for a while. This shows how observation and empirical evidence is just as important in scientific research as laboratory findings.

We have to observe the karma and analyze it empirically before we can take it to the next level and master it experimentally. In many cases we would never even make it into the laboratory without somebody reporting unusual and compelling observations in their environments. This was the case with Uri Geller's mother observing the spoon break which opened the door for all of his research. Stella Crenshaw reported to price that she observed amazing telekinetic effects in her environment which gave rise to their research. Palladino at an early age noticed empirically that she had some kind of paranormal powers. In my own case, I observed amazing telekinetic phenomenon happening in my environment with refrigerators, the whereabouts of others, the weather, the functioning on cars, and cellular phones and much more.

Estebany has always been quite eager to cooperate with scientists and discover more about his amazing talents. Grad's first experiment with Estabany involved healing Goiters (enlarged thyroids) on mice with PK. In this experiment, seventy mice were induced with Goiters through dietary methods. The experimental group of mice received healing treatment from Estebany, one control group received no treatment, and another group was placed into a cage to reproduce the temperature from Estebany's hands.

The thyroids of both control groups increased in size significantly faster than the group being treated by Estebany's PK. In a similar experiment, Estebany simply treated pieces of wool and cotton with his PK healing force that were placed into the experimental cages. In the two control cages, he placed similar untreated materials. Again, the results showed a markedly slower growth rate in goiters on mice within the experimental group that received the treated pieces of wool and cotton.

Grad's most famous experiments involved anesthetized mice that were treated with PK to heal wounded skin. In one of these experiments, mice were first anesthetized and small sections of the skin were removed from their backs. Precise measurements of the size of each wound was made by covering the wound with transparent plastic and tracing its outline onto the plastic. The outline was then transferred onto paper and cut out. The pieces of paper for each group of mice were weighed on a highly sensitive balance scale.

The mice were divided into three groups. The group labeled E was treated by Estebany's PK, two times per day for fifteen minutes, five days per week and once on Saturdays. While not being treated, the mice were held in ordinary laboratory cages. The second group of mice, the control batch, were not treated by Estebany at all. However, they were transferred to cages that were heated to reproduce the temperature emitted on the experimental group by Estebany's hand. This transfer also subjected them to the same amount of stress as the experimental group, which was also transferred into other cages.

Another group was also untreated by Estabany, but when they were in the treatment cages, the cages were slightly heated to replicate the heat transferred on the experimental cage by Estebany's hands. The scientists then measured the wounds of the mice in all cages on the first, eleventh, and fourteenth days after wounding. On the day following the wounding and the day thereafter, no significant differences were observed in any of the three groups. On the eleventh day, there was little difference noticed between the control group and the heated groups, but the wounds on the E group were much smaller than those in both of the control groups. By the fourteenth day, the wounds of most of the E group had totally healed to the size of a pinpoint. However, the wounds of both untreated groups were significantly larger. Dr. Grad has replicated this experiment and obtained similar results.

In 1971 at the Parapsychological Convention in Durham, North Carolina, Anita Watkins reported another ingenious experimental approach for using mice in PK healing research. They measured the speed at which mice that were labeled "healed" and "unhealed" regained consciousness after being placed under anesthesia in etherizers. In each trial, two mice were used, one in the experimental group that was treated with PK, and one in the control group that was not.

A previously selected and randomly generated number determined whether the first mice to loose consciousness would be selected from the experimental or control group. Then, a healer attempted to treat the mice. His effort was considered successful, if those mice recovered consciousness before the ones in the control group that were untreated. In these laboratory trials, the results were considered positive. The mice who received the healing energies recovered from anesthesia much faster then the ones in the control group. This study is quite peculiar because not all of the people involved with healing the mice claimed to be healers. Some of the participants were just members of the staff at the Institute of Parapsychology.

At the next PA Convention, Elendur Haraldson of the ASPR and Thorsteinn Thorsteinsson from the University of Iceland reported on their PK experiments involving yeast. They mixed yeast and nutritive solution, before subjecting half of the 20 tubes to a ten-minute treatment by a healer who was not allowed to touch them. All 20 tubes were then stored for twenty-four hours, and then they were measured by a light-absorbency test. Twelve sessions were conducted using eleven healers. The scores were slightly positive.

Out of 120 pairs of test tubes, 58 showed more growth in the experimental tubes. 33 showed less growth, 29 tubes showed an equal amount of growth that were subjected to the healers touch. The most striking aspect of this study was that three of the seven subjects were responsible for nearly all of the PK effects. These three individuals all had a background in healing. Two of them were "mental healers," and the other was an ordinary medical doctor.

Another experiment in this area was conducted in 1958 where Nigel Richmond conducted experiments in England concerning the effects of PK on biological systems. He placed a drop of pond water under a microscope and then watched the paramecia, which live in the water swim around. Richmond divided the water drop into four quadrants. He then willed for the paramecia to travel into one of the segments. He randomly selected the target quarter (where he wanted the paramecia to swim) for each trial.

Each trial lasted fifteen seconds. During this time he would select a temporally immobile paramecia and will it to swim in a particular direction. 1495 trials were conducted and they were all extremely successful. This convinced Richmond that he can actually influenced the behavior of single celled animals through the power of his will. While this study does not specifically pertain to healing, it does prove that telekinesis functions at a microscopic level to affect biological systems. This kind of biological influenced can be related to healing, which also takes place on a microscopic level.

Sri Pranananda reported to me that a friend of his used a psychotronics device to charge ponds of water on his catfish farm. The laboratory results were striking. Ponds were clear and not nearly as muddy as before the water optimizing device was used to charge it. Eighty percent of the fish survived during the experimental phase, while eighty percent perished during the control phase where no psychotronic apparatus was used. So, they had double harvests and the experimenters felt that the quality of the fish meat was significantly better.

Now, I must use this juncture to reiterate that we should avoid eating meat according to the scriptures of transcendental yoga. Many people are not aware that even fish does indeed qualify as meat! However, I consider it the most acceptable form of meat if one *needs* to eat it. For example, Jesus himself fed a large flock lots of fish meat when they were in need of food through a powerful display of his PK where he multiplied to food for the masses. However, there is dissent concerning whether he actually ate the fish.

While I do hold vegetarianism as the highest spiritual standard, I also know that there are times when it is necessary to eat meat. In those times, I admonish my disciples and readers to simply eat a little bit of fish, but avoid cow meat totally. The cow is one of the most sacred creatures in the universe, and they should be protected and respected by all means! Cows are treasured by Lord Sri Krsna, who was a cowherd boy worshiped by the gopis (cowherd girls). This represents God's intimate and loving transcendental bond with the cows who dwell with Him in Krsnaloka. In fact, the scriptures reveal to us that there are entire oceans of cow milk in the spiritual world! This phenomenon shows us how cows are very spiritually elevated creatures that are too be revered and protected. Hence, the Vedic yogic scriptures tell us that whoever kills a cow will be sentenced to rebirth in the punishing material world, just as many times as there are hairs on the cows entire body! Moreover, the scriptures teach us that in some future life, that animal will have a body that is suitable to kill its murderers. What undesirable punishments. If one is guilty of these offenses against Krsna, then I admonish one to immediately turn to His Lotus Feet and surrender for forgiveness. Before the Lord descended to this planet 5000 years ago, the Earth was being overrun by demons who had assumed physical bodies.

It was a very dangerous time on the planet mainly because the principles of real religion severely deteriorated similar to modern times. That polluted atmosphere gave rise to the monumental Battle of Kuruksetra. At that time, the presiding deity (demigod) of the earth who was a cow personally visited Lord Sri Krsna in His Abode of Krsnaloka to plead for His most divine intervention. That was when God decided to incarnate in His original "*Syamasundara* form," according to the yogic scriptures. Cows nourish our planet, while protecting our health with delights such as yogurt, butter, cheese, ghee and milk. Many scientists contend that global warming is partially attributed to excessive consumption of red meat. Apparently, this this destruction of cows is affecting the balance of our whole ecosystem.

A spectacular test involving the connection between PK and biology was conducted by Jean Barry M.D. in 1968 who carried out his experiments in cooperation with the staff at the Institute of Agronomy in Broudoux France. Rather than working with animal life, Barry studied the effects of PK on fungus cultures. Pitri dishes containing the cultures were prepared a day prior to the experiment and placed in an environment where they could thrive. The following day, the subjects were each given ten dishes.

The subjects concentrated on five of the cultures in an attempt to stifle growth using their PK. The remaining five dishes left as the controls, and no effort to impede growth was made on them. Eleven subjects submitted to the study, and a total of thirty nine trials were conducted. After measuring the experimental and control fungus culture, Barry found that his subjects were able to mentally inhibit the growth of the fungus they focused on.

Dr. Grad has also contributed immensely to the field of PK, by providing irrefutable scientific proof that PK and will power can effect plant growth. Again, early in his career, Grad worked closely with Wilhelm Reich. In Grad's experiments with plants, he also worked with Estebany, who treated seedlings that were experimentally injured by a mild saline solution. Estebany held the saline solution in hand, before it was poured onto the experimental group. He did not make any contact with the flask of saline that was poured onto the seedlings in the control group. Blind measurements indicated markedly better plant growth for the flask that Estebany held.

In a similar experiment, Grad used three different subjects. He experimented with a man described as having a "green thumb," a depressive neurotic, and a depressive psychotic. Plants watered from the flask held by the man with the green thumb grew much faster than control plants. Those watered by the neurotic grew slightly faster than usual, and those watered by the psychotic grew much slower. Other studies have been conducted, where subjects attempt to influence the electrical activity of one of two plants in front of them. Blind scoring of the results showed more changes in the plants that subjects tried to mentally influence by PK than in the others. This data suggests that changes in plant physiology resulting from a person's intent might be attributed to the person's PK.

Dr. Grad has also discovered that PK can foster fermentation increase in yeast. All four experiments he conducted in this area have produced phenomenal PK effects. This is consistent with the findings of French researchers, who discovered that subjects attempting to inhibit the growth of fungus by PK were successful. Grad's work with Estebany certainly evidences some connection between PK and healing in living organisms. Estebany was also involved to take part in experiments conducted by Sister Justa Smith, an enzymologist who was from Rosary Hill College in Buffallo. N.Y. For her research, she used solutions of trypson, which is a digestive enzyme.

For each day of the experiment, a portion of the solution was divided into four parts that were placed into separate containers. The first stopper flask was treated by Estebany for roughly 75 minutes. The second sample was exposed to ultraviolet light, which retards activity of tripson, and a third flask was placed in a high magnetic field. The fourth flask was a control and it was heated to reach the same temperature as the healers hands, but otherwise it was not subjected to any changes. Sister Justa found at the end of her experiment that the flasks treat by Estebany increased in trypsin activity just as much as exposure to a magnetic field of 13,000 gauss. By the way, the magnetic field of the Earth itself is only about 0.5 gauss.

Chapter 8: Introducing the Fridge Phenomenon (FP)

The Fridge Phenomenon (FP) is distinct electrokinetic feat, where I am unquestionably able to remotely control the functioning of nearly all refrigerator units, by causing them to turn on or off. The FP is triggered by my mental impulses, thoughts, emotions, speech, bodily movements, my direct will and use of *psychotronic technologies*. I discovered this phenomenon while studying as an international law student in Holland. The FP began happening shortly after my Dutch Guru, Bhakta Michael, initiated me into transcendental science of Bhakti Yoga and gave me two Vedic Power Mantras. One of the most fascinating things about the FP is that it can act totally on its own and independent of my will, yet I am clearly able to control the phenomenon. At times I can literally feel the PK Force from my body controlling the refrigerator like a powerful magnetic electromagnetic energy. I have determined that PK Force obviously has its own highly intelligent properties, it can certainly "think for itself," and act on its own volition. It knows what we are doing and thinking so it is certainly of the divine, cosmic and celestial nature from another world. It is controlled by the thoughts. Again, the FP is just something that works on its own like most other psi phenomenon. And, whatever arises from that which works also is viable. On the other hand, something that arises out of that which does not work is doomed to failure, like fruits from a poisonous tree. All ideas, thought and courses of action that are born out of an invalid idea are also dysfunctional.

In this life, we are all desperately in need of finding that magical something/anything that actually works. The wise man builds his house upon the rock (that which really works) and the foolish man buildt his house upon the sand (that which does not work). What will the foolish man do when the rain comes tumbling down? We can not ever forget that the FP was discovered only as a direct result of yogic devotional service unto Lord Sri Krsna who has *always been* the only solid rock! There will be those who are only concerned with challenging the FP for one reason or another, which is analogous to shooting themselves in the foot. That is rather unfortunate because these "Doubting Thomases" will never have the benefits in this life or the next of viable philosophies, theories and breakthroughs that are based on the FP discovery. Please note that all it takes is one grain of sand to destroy an entire engine in an automobile. Similarly, all that it takes is one viable idea or thought to change the whole fate of humanity. Therefore, we should use the stark reality of the FP to approach life itself from a whole new perspective--in a whole new age. The FP has shown me that as a telekinetic spiritualistic medium that I am able to effortlessly channel the power of Lord Sri Krsna and bring it right here.

Vaishnavas generally follow a process of initiation known as *Diksha*, administered by a guru, who trains them in order to understand Vaishnava practices. At the time of initiation the disciples are given a specific mantra, which is repeated, either out loud or just within the mind, as a form of worship to Vishnu or one of His "Avatars." This form of repetitious prayer is known as Japa. This process of receiving initiation and training from a spiritual master is premised on injunctions within sacred yogic scriptures in Vaishnava traditions. Along these lines the scriptures provide:

"Just try to learn the truth by approaching a spiritual master. Inquire from him submissively and render service unto him. The self-realized souls can impart knowledge unto you because they have seen the truth."(Bhagavad-Gita)

"One who is initiated into the Vaishnava mantra and who is devoted to worshiping Lord Vishnu is a Vaishnava. One who is devoid of these practices is not a Vaishnava."(Padma Purana) [8]

On the other hand, other scriptures (in this instance from the Gaudiya lineage) explain that: *"Who chants the holy name of Krishna just once may be considered a Vaishnava. Such a person is worshipable and is the topmost human being.."*(Chaitanya Charitamrita)

Shortly after I received Diksha from Bhakta Michael and began practicing this royal mantra yoga, I began to observe highly paranormal effects happening with the small refrigerator at my home in Amsterdam. In the final analysis, I am only able to wield this kind of control over material nature because of the complexities of my karma. I believe that this energy is manifesting in this way to help people overcome the greatest challenges and obstacles in life. As you will see, this electrokinetic propensity of mine is not limited to affecting refrigerators!

For me, the FP provides concrete proof that thought energy/thought forms directly control the physical world. And that can be a scary thought. Many people have been seeking some example of true PK all of their lives, and some will search for their whole lives to find it. It is only the most auspicious of Karma in this information *age* that exposes the stark reality of FP to the most fortunate soul searchers. For those that are deluded by the spirit of doubt, I admonish you to fix this problem by seeking the face of God before it is too late to save yourself from damnation.

So many people ask me "why the refrigerator? My answer is that I do not know because my consciousness is finite. We all know so very little about ultimate reality because our consciousness is limited. However, Lord Sri Krsna is recognized by the greatest spiritual masters, the most adept sages, and the highest yogis as God Himself, as He has supreme consciousness as the "Super Soul" (*paramatma*) that lives within everybody's heart! He is the well of all power, knowledge and intelligence. We are also limited in our ability to control matters in our lives. However, Lord Sri Krsna is known as the "Supreme Controller," as He controls everything and everybody, including the most powerful demigods such as Lord Bhamaji and Lord Siva. Furthermore, we are all limited in our capacity to enjoy anything and everything. Conversely, God is known as the "Supreme Enjoyer" because his capacity to enjoy is limitless and infinite.

When we render homage and service unto Him, He is naturally pleased and enjoys it. Many people wonder why their prayers are never answered. This is a great question for a Guruji! Prayers are often not answered because we fail to recognize that it is not God's constitutional position is not to serve man. It is our constitutional position to serve the Creator. When we do that, then he always reciprocates. That is how is discovered the Fridge Phenomenon. Make no mistake about it. Of course, the next logical question is how are we to please God. In order to please Him, you have to make an adequate sacrifice or offering. The lord Clearly says in Srimad Bhagavad-gita that if we are to offer a leaf, a flower or fruit unto

Him, then he will accept it as "the pious offering of the pure in heart." According to the Great Spiritual Master Srila Prabhupada, the most perfect sacrifice is the repetitious chanting of the Lord's Holy Names, which is the Maha Mantra.

This is all confirmed and revealed within the world's most authoritative yogic scriptures. Pleasing Lord Sri Krsna is the most critical survival skill that you will ever learn. And, do not forget that survival is the central purpose of all yoga by definition. The Lord is especially pleased when we sacrifice, by engaging our minds and intelligence in meditating on His transcendental information. Unfortunately in this age of Kali, most people are not enjoying life to the fullest because they don't have what they want or need. That is because it is not our constitutional right to enjoy anything at all! All of our enjoyment is a privilege that must be first sanctioned by the Hand of God. So, when we first please Him through the royal yogic practice of Bhakti, then He always reciprocates us with the highest benefits of enjoying life on all levels. The FP was a gift directly from God in my greatest time of spiritual need. He knows perfectly well that I enjoy being able to produce this feat constantly. God knows perfectly well that I enjoy having many other telekinetic and electrokinetic abilities that he has blessed me with. This yogic science of enjoying life can be explained even better through the following analogy:

Suppose that pleasure represents a rope that you keep tugging on because you naturally want more of it. The more slack that the rope gives you, the more pleasure you have in life. Krsna is the one grasping the other end of that rope, and He will not give you any slack unless He is sufficiently pleased. That is why success, happiness and enjoyment in life is purely a spiritual matter. Look around you and consider how many people that you know are actually enjoying life to the fullest. Unfortunately, its getting harder to find enjoyment everyday on planet Earth. The material scientists even predict that enjoyment on this planet is quickly diminishing for most forms of life and especially humanity. Now, consider how many people that you know are making an earnest effort everyday to please God Himself, Lord Sri Krsna.

Again, you will probably find it hard to spot such an individual. This is the yogic concept for enjoying life to the fullest. I have a disciple who periodically attends Rainbow Gatherings, which are held at various locations around the world. He tells me that for some strange reason, he has experienced the most enjoyment and pleasure at the gatherings where the Vaishnava devotees are chanting incessantly! That is because when we chant Hare Krsna, God is very satisfied and pleased, which brings everyone in the whole area the greatest spiritual pleasure! Since everything in existence is actually spiritual, pleasure is experienced on the highest levels through by service and devotion to God. Hence, Krsna Consciousness is the highest form of public service.

The more He is pleased with our service and worship, the more all of our problems begin to melt away right before our eyes. Moreover, the yogic merging process between our soul and the supreme enjoyer causes us to enjoy everything in life on a blissful transcendental level. Suicide, drug abuse, depression, and many other serious personal afflictions are only a result of not enjoying life! Pretentious attitudes, fascism, inflated egos, and superiority complexes of any kind are the highest indications of a fool, as Krsna is the one who decides who sinks and who swims! In the final analysis, God is the only one that decides who is the highest, and what He bestows upon us, He can also take right back in the blinking of an eye! Many nations around the world, for example, are figuring that out the hard way.

When Lord Sri Krsna is protecting you, then there is nothing can hurt you, and if Krsna wants to destroy you, then there is nothing in the world that can save you. So the real task in this human form of life is to determine factually what pleases God Himself (Krsna), and then to perpetually live out that Dharma. The Lord thoroughly explains how to practice the highest yogic process for pleasing Him in Srimad *Bhagavad-Gita*. This sublime yogic process will certainly foster the specific kinds of changes that you are seeking in life. It is a fact. What a merciful blessing from the Lord!

We can see how Krsna consciousness is all about connecting with God on a very personal level. Clearly, the FP (the main subject of this chapter) is a very personable manifestation of God. Since just about everybody has a refrigerator, and knows hoe they function, Krsna is manifesting in a way that we all can connect with in this specific time. Without these kinds of *signs and wonders*, many people would never be able to develop the faith that is necessary to make it back to Him in the spiritual skies; many people could not make the types of psychological connections that are necessary for internalizing God's existence as a highly active controller.

Since Lord Sri Krsna always reciprocates us for worshipping Him with love, devotion and affection, anything can happen in our lives when we serve Him. I am living proof. When God is pleased with our activities, then our karma is positively, permanently, and commensurately changed at the core. The Hand of God dictates what happens to us in life and the specific kind of fruit that our trees bear. That is the secret to life and the reason why the FP is happening here on earth right now. We could speculate for the rest of this whole life about what is causing the FP. Remember that PK is only a label for something that the scientist still can not fully apprehend. However, the imperishable science of God has all of the answers that we need to understand these kinds of paranormal feats, and to produce even greater miracles in the name of Jagannatha ("Lord of the Universe"). That is exactly why I discovered the FP at the exact same point when I first started bhakti mantra practice.

Naturally, this discovery has opened great doors, and brought me blessing that I had not imagined or planned for. Anybody can witness the same kind of personal and spiritual transformation, by simply surrendering right now to the Primaeval Lord named Hari. Upon surrendering to the Lotus Feet of the supersoul, *anybody can* experience the most phenomenal spiritual blessings and PK effects. Of this there is no doubt! This goes to show you how worship and service unto the Supreme Personality of Godhead is the key to fulfilment in our lives, enlightenment and self actualization. It is the highest road to achievement, self help, self-sufficiency, happiness and success. It is the most powerful way of developing a mind that is transcendental for controlling material nature and its forces. All skeptics should first recognize that they are foolish for doubting the capability of God's almighty hand. They also have an insurmountable battle to win in disproving my evidence for the existence of the FP and its intrinsic connection with yoga. It is not possible for critics to succeed in convincing me or any of the eye witnesses to the FP that we are mistaken.

The story behind my relationship with Bhakta Michael is quite fascinating. As soon as I got off of the plane for my relocation into Amsterdam, he picked me up in a random cab and escorted me to my new home. He never mentioned anything about being a yogi, and we did not discuss it, until I he helped me to move three months later. When we first met, he merely helped me get acquainted with the city. He never mentioned anything about being involved with yoga and we did not discuss it at all. After Bhakta Michael dropped me off at my new place, he gave me his business card and told me to call anytime. I got so busy that I had no chance to speak with him again, until I suddenly and unexpectedly needed to move into a new place on the other end of the town

I had nobody else to call for help in relocating, so I called him for assistance. Although I do have a strong background with Hare Krsna, I was inactive as a devotee for a long time. After I met this Guru, I fortuitously stumbled upon a small book entitled *Easy Journey to Other Planets*, By Srila Prabhupada, which helped me to renew my divine consciousness. As I read this little book, I felt my divine mind expanding int the cosmos and my true identity being restored. So, I started practicing the regulative principles. However, I was not active with japa, until he gave me the maha mantra.

As we were discussing mundane matters as he helped me move, the subject somehow shifted to metaphysics and meditation. I told him about my involvements with this new form of yoga based on finding the book. At that point, I learned that he has practiced *bhakti-yoga* for more than ten years. He immediately knew that the book I found was written by Srila Prabhupada, even though I was unsure who wrote it. He told me about his pilgrimages throughout India and interactions with Vaishnavas there. He helped me renew my divine consciousness and we both witnessed many miracles including the FP immediately after meeting.

The FP highlights the increasing integration of Eastern and Western ways of life. It was born from a marriage between Eastern transcendental thought on one hand, and the heart of Western-mechanistic science, culture and technology on the other. Along those lines, the FP provides an entirely new way of studying, observing and proving the stark reality of PK. It is a classic psi manifestation that substantiates the reality of mind over matter.

The recorded instances of the FP that I provide in the next chapter are intended to help the reader make sense of this PK effect; to further your understanding of this intelligent force, and how it functions in the most accurate light. Another distinct advantage of these empirical records is that they expose neophytes in transcendental yoga and metaphysics to fundamental occult practices, perspectives tools and concepts. This gives readers a jump start in creating the ideal spiritual life on any level of their choice, while making an informed decision. It also enables you to analyze this energy and how it functions in a way that is easy to understand and even entertaining! Most importantly, it exposes the mind to real metaphysical and yogic practice in action that has proven its power. Each of the recorded instances illustrates the supernatural PK force at work, and helps us better understand how it controls matter.

Again, the FP was initially observed when I began chanting the mantras supplied to me by Bhakta Michael. I first noticed that quite often my refrigerator would turn on or off at the very same exact second that I began chanting. It is an extreme form of synchronicity! Other times, as soon as I would start to chant, the refrigerator would shut down and loose all power in an instant, just as if I pulled its plug. Of course, I could not help but to notice this, but at first I acted oblivious and ignored it because the mere thought of it seemed unfathomable to me at the time and even a bit scary. I believe that electrokinesis is a distinct frequency that connects the minds directly to the whole world of electricity on a psychic level! Clearly the mind can control electricity which is evidenced by the FP and other phenomenon related to lights. So, imagine having the ability to unconsciously control the whole world of electricity at some level. Of course, much of our whole modern world functions on electricity. That could explain the very high degree over material nature as a whole that the electrokinetic person can wield.

We can not forget that the human body and animals also function on electricity. Many parapsychologists believe that our "astral bodies" are also heavily affected by electricity. That belief stems from reports of near-death victims, who claim to have been stuck to electric wires during the time they were presumed dead. Since so much in our existence is intrinsically interrelated with electricity both inside and outside of our bodies, I believe that the electrokinetic mind is the key top superhuman existence. In fact, it is one of the highest mystical powers that The Lord can bestow upon his unalloyed devotee who is engaged in His divine yogic service. For example, electrokinesis greatly amplifies ones magical powers on all levels, and ones psi abilities because if one can control electricity then one can control what is outside of his body with ease.

The electrical impulses outside of the body form a vast infinite network of energy that the electrokinetic mind can control at any distance. Since electricity and thought can apparently work hand-in hand, electrokinesis also accounts for all action at a distance. A classic example of this is bi-location phenomenon or the ability to influence the physical locations of others. How in the world in that possible? Well, electrokinesis is a powerful framework for understanding how that all works. Human bodies run on electricity and thought at both the unconscious and conscious level. If the "EK'er" is able to affect the electricity with his mind, then electrical impulses in the bodies, brain waves and even the thoughts of there also may be affected. All that I can do is report to you in sheer honestly about what it takes to develop electrokinesis, which will indeed catapult your whole life to a whole new *level*. My advise is to serve Lord Sri Krana and to worship Him with all of your heart.

However, I understand that many of my readers will not accept that advice. So I have provided other ways for you to connected with PK, telekinesis and electrokinetic power. You will find it in the chapter on telekinetic triggers.

Like many of the scientists from the Victorian era, I simply ignored this PK phenomenon (The FP) until I no longer could! On one occasion, I began chanting and at the exact same second I started, I got a cell phone call from Bhakta Michael. I then told him that the FP was happening, and he was absolutely amazed. He had never heard of anything like it before. The most amazing thing about this phenomenon is that it happens constantly without me ever having to attempt. Most of the time, it feels like some intelligent force within me makes it happen totally outside of my control! Whether I make the FP happen willingly or inadvertently, it is a fascinating experience because it represents the essence of my mystical powers and spirituality.

I indeed have the ability to control refrigerators by directly commanding them to turn on or off. Refrigerator units of all types and styles, including vending machines and even water fountains are instantly triggered to turn on and off by my telekinetic powers. Many times, they react as soon as approach them, when I enter into the area, when I walk past them, and especially when I make any physical contact with them. As you will read, sometimes as soon as I touch the refrigerator, or make any physical contact with it even accidentally, the unit instantly turns on or off at the exact same split second. This also has been noticed by many employees within certain grocery stores that I patronize. My ability to unconsciously produce this effect is one of the reasons why the FP was discovered while I was not looking for it. This feeling of "eureka" or "I found it" is the most powerful experiences in any discovery and in this human form of life.

The FP demonstrates that what we see with the naked eye is only an inferior form of energy. What we perceive with the five senses is like in a dream that is controlled by the transcendental mind. This is the reasoning behind all transcendental meditation (TM) practice and philosophy. Of course in the Western world after so much knowledge of the highest TM becomes available, we should expect to witness miracles of all forms manifesting in our most advanced technologies such as cell phones, automobiles, computers and refrigerators. Here you will learn about how this magnificent PK force has affected all of kinds of technologies in my environment.

The main object of this book is to explore how we all can use this same transcendental life force to change karma. The FP follows me wherever I go, others easily notice it, and I have certainly learned to control it. However, I do not enjoy controlling my PK for amusement purposes, as it creates an unbearable sense of tension and even great emotional pain and stress. Since this is a well established case of true PK, I am now building upon the framework of the FP, and its far-reaching implications for all.I have repeatedly conducted controlled experiments, where I intentionally   trigger the FP to confirm its existence. Based on countless trials and extensive empirical research, I have proved through the FP that mind over matter is totally real. I never knew it was so real until this phenomenon jumped right out at me and changed my entire life. Most people never have this kind of thing happen to them, as true PK is one of the rarest forms of psychic phenomenon. So, it is critical for me to present the FP to the world in this handbook as a new scientific mind over matter discovery. We should be principally concerned with the extent of its implications.

After proving the reality of the FP through the experimental and empirical research approaches that you will read about in the following chapters, I decided not to waste anymore of my time and energy playing around with refrigerators. Moreover, my Sri Pranananda admonished me to move on, and to develop my powers even further. He assured me that these abilities were not limited to the refrigerator. The difference between this handbook and many others on mind over matter or PK is that I provide very practical and effective approaches for integrating this powerful force into your lives.

Many other paranormal cases involving *synchronicity* precipitated my discovery of the FP. Again, this mainly started in my life after I met Bhakta Michael, which activated my shaktipat kundalini energy. I first noticed that something uncanny was going on when I was at a cross walk in Amsterdam. I noticed a lady also preparing to cross standing directly across the street from me. We walked right past each other, and I proceeded to my home on the other end of town. I stayed home for several hours and then went into the city to place a call at a random international call center. As I was waiting at the call center counter waiting to be addressed by the clerk, I looked to my left and saw the very same lady that was at the crosswalk standing beside me. That felt a little startling, sort of like something that would happen in a horror movie or the *Twilight Zone*! Of course I noticed it but just ignored it and chalked it up to a "coincidence." This same kind of phenomenon persisted until I could no longer ignore it.

On another occasion, I was on my way to an office to handle some business. On the way there while riding my bike, I stopped another crosswalk. Right in front of me, I noticed there were two women paired up on a bike. One was riding on the back holding a bag that said "Gimmicks," which is a chain store in Holland. I proceeded to the office far on the other end of town, where it took several hours to handle my business. After I left the office several hours later, I took random streets beside winding canals, to get back home. Far from where I first saw these ladies at the stop light, and far from the office, these same two women on the same bike rode right in front of me out of nowhere. I was riding home at a very fast speed taking random streets and avenues when they reappeared.

On another occasion, I was having a meeting with a group of friends. After we were finished meeting, I rode home on my bike, and on the way there I saw two kids with quite fancy bikes pull right in front of me. About thirty minutes later, I was in a totally different area of town far away, and these same two boys suddenly reappeared again right next to me. I noticed this and was very confused, but again I ignored it just like I first ignored the FP. However, one of the teenagers actually started to panic and insisted that I was following them. I assured him that they were not being followed and that this same phenomenon has been persistently happening to me.

Since one of them also was baffled by this and fairly shocked, I considered that as proof of this mystical physical location phenomenon. They are both eye witnesses. I told them about other cases involving this form of synchronicity. The other youth said that he has also had some experiences with this phenomenon and was very confused by all of it. He told me about specific times where it has also happened to him in the city and took him by surprise. Since they both were amazed, and even claimed that I was following them, I knew that my hunch about influencing the physical whereabouts of others were valid and not "delusions." This also suggests that my other observations in the realm of PK are valid, particularly where there are eye witnesses and neutral observers who have openly corroborated it.

On another occasion, I was walking home and noticed a man who definitely resembled a mythical character. Several hours later, I was in another area of town and saw him again at a random location. A liberal English Muslim saint became one of my spiritual advisors and Reiki therapist in Amsterdam. Shortly after we began became acquainted, we both noticed fortuitously encountering each other far more frequently than chance or "coincidence" could ever account for. I asked her if this happens with other people, and she assured me that it does not. She is a powerful Reiki therapist indeed because I have always suffered from jaw problems and one day, she treated me with Reiki. The very next day, my entire jaw worked differently and there was a lot of grinding I could hear when I moved it. Clearly her treatment triggered something extreme in my jaw muscle. She predicted that the grinding in my jaw bone would go away after a Fe days that it had to adjust. She was right, and its now totally healed.

Even after I moved back to North America, I noticed this physical location synchronicity happening with several people in the community. One person named Alex became a disciple and is still so confused about why he encounters me much more frequently than anybody else he knows. He even said to me, "I never run into people this often and this is very weird. I don't know how this is possible!" One time, I purchased a beautiful statue of Lord Sri Krsna from a local metaphysical store that was having a sale. Right after purchasing the statue, I placed it inside of my bag and proceeded to the transit station in town. On the way there I saw Alex walking on the other side of the street. After waiting at the station for a while, I got on a random bus, and sure enough Alex just happened to get on the very same bus a few minutes after I boarded.

He said "wait a minute, I just saw you on the other side of town walking on the opposite side of the street, and we somehow happened to get on the same bus?" I told him that I had the Krsna idol in my bag, which I believe triggered PK. We started having a discussion about Tibetan Buddhist ideas, which was a convenient way of helping him to make sense of this phenomenon However, the best way of understanding how this works is to recognize that this active transcendental energy is all powerful, controlling and intelligent, which accounts for this mystical physical location phenomenon.

I once had a co-worker and we extensively discussed transcendental yoga. On one occasion, months after we stopped working together, I was chanting various mystical mantras and performing *kriyas* in the woods for about an hour. Note that I hardly ever go into the woods and do this. I just got bored one day and decided to take a walk down there. Out of nowhere, right after I was finished with this intense spiritual work, I mysteriously encountered him, just as I was walking out of the wooded park area. This experience indicates how the high level of PK energy that I was generating in this yogic session somehow took control over material affairs. Once again, the energy apparently had an affect on physical whereabouts.. When we bumped into each other, I told him that I just got done chanting in the park for about an hour. He admitted that it was highly unusual, as we never see each other around and that was the only time it has ever happened. The precise timing and location of the encounter indicates that some intelligent energetic force was summoned and manifested this mind over matter effect.

The fact that I do not try to trigger the FP does not affect its frequency or consistency. Refraining from attempt to perform even makes it happen more persistently and intensively. On the other hand, I do find it fun to direct my PK for some specific purposes, such as influencing events, for weather/storm control, for self-improvement, chakra conditioning and karmic restructuring. Apparently, I can trigger nearly any refrigerator to turn on or off by using my PK. Note that there are two kinds of refrigerators: One model always stays running. However, most people have refrigerators that randomly turn on and off, which have no timers to control the random on-off cycles.

For me, the FP is an excellent way to work with mind over matter and test how it functions. I know that many others will find it as a useful point of reference and example of a true mind over matter effect. Whatever energy is involved with causing the FP is affecting what actually *happens in reality*. I have noticed that after clearing the chakras with PK energy one by one through meditation or using psychotronics, the FP becomes even more intensified! In other words, I can intensify all PK phenomenon I produce at will. The FP then becomes even much more controlled by my unconscious mind, thought processes, and random bodily movements.

While it is important not to jump to conclusions or assume anything, it is equally important not to overlook this energy when we sense it manifesting something like this on the physical plane. Most people are concerned about how the FP is relevant to life as a whole. I have found that this energy is certainly not limited to controlling the fridge. By releasing psychotronic power and directing it to do one thing or another, one immediately learns that life itself can be influenced and even controlled with PK just like a dream! That is why the secret doctrines of Tibetan Buddhism confirm that the dream and waking states of consciousness are non different and merely opposite sides of the same pole of consciousness. Both levels of consciousness are controlled by the mind. Note that even in the dream state, it is often difficult to wield control of what happens! Most of have had dreams where we could not control anything!

The illusory nature of the whole material world becomes even more apparent when using PK consciously within the context of yoga.

After I moved back to North America from Holland, this rather unique paranormal phenomenon followed me right into my new home! The refrigerator in the place that I moved to was highly responsive to my PK. It did not only react to my chanting or speech, which was initially the case. I noticed that it was clearly being directly triggered to turn on or off by my bodily movements, thoughts, and other activities. When I moved out of this place, the next refrigerator I had was so sensitive to my PK that it broke down only about two weeks after I moved in. It had to be totally replaced. The next refrigerator they brought in was no less sensitive to my PK.

After a long time of very obvious psychic phenomenon in the home within my refrigerator, which my grandmother also observed, she became very concerned about it, and encouraged me to start documenting these accounts. To illustrate the complex nature of the FP, one day I called my grandmother using a calling card. As soon as she picked up the phone and said "hello," my refrigerator turned on at the exact same second. This is an example of how the energy behind the FP morphs in highly intelligent ways. Of course, I told her what just happened. Then about an hour later, my calling card suddenly ran out of time, and we were disconnected without warning in the middle of the conversation. I called her back without using the calling card, on my regular phone line. Again, when she picked up the phone and said "hello" for the second time, my fridge turned on instantly. This is what I call the phone phenomenon, where my PK clearly affects phones of all varieties.

During one conversation with my grandmother, I began explaining to her how I am constantly noticing an excessive number of cars in my environment with one front light this is not working! Based on her deeply spiritual background, she knows a lot about these kinds of paranormal issues happening with yoga. However, she never heard of anything like this or the FP before. This car light phenomenon is happening so frequently in my presence that many other people who are with me also notice it. In other words, they are being subjected to my individualized karmic powers in the objective world. Some people have commented that this only happens when they are with me. On one occasion, I was telling my grandmother about this car light phenomenon, and she became really confused about what it means. During this conversation, we observed no less than five cars right outside of my window that had one front light blown out! They just kept driving up one after the next! Whether or not you choose to believe in this car-light phenomenon has no bearing on the truth. Many people have witnessed it for themselves, and have been quite shocked at how it works. Really, it is nothing but another classic case of electrokinesis coupled with psychokinesis. That's is, the ability to both affect the electrical functioning of cars and there whereabouts with the mind and specifically the thoughts.

Interestingly enough, there is a post office across from where I live where I observe a great number of these front-light afflicted cars. I constantly notice an excessive amount of cars coming out of the parking lot or driving past the post office with one front light that is not working. Sometimes it happens so much that it leaves me utterly bewildered. Sometimes, one car right after the next drives out of the parking lot with one front light that is not working. It began happening so much that I decided something spiritual at that post office must be causing this. However, it is not limited to the post office, this is happening everywhere in my environment.

Even the biggest "doubting Thomases" that I know are directly subjected to it. One time I was with friend in a rural mountainous area, and we both saw a car with the front light blown out. That was when I confided to him my psychokinetic track record for attracting cars like this in my environment. He immediately began to challenge and resist it overtly, but at the very same time I showed him another car at the stop sign a few feet to our right that also had one front like not working. Even though some may say this is a coincidence, there is ample evidence to show that this is a specific pattern connected with a telekinetic mind. It is obviously nothing for such a mind to affect electronic technologies at a distance. We have already seen many examples of this. Another time I was with a friend of mine from Africa and I explained to him how this car-light phenomenon works with me. He seemed a bit skeptical at first, until we witnessed two cars drive right past us, both having one front lightbulb that was not working. The most fascinating thing about this is that it happening most, even with eye witnesses, after intensive chanting of the Maha Mantra or discussing matters related to Sri Krsna. That is also the case with the Fridge Phenomenon.

On many occasions, these cars are all around me. I finally realized after thinking about this post office issue that my good friend from India works there who is also a Guru! I think that this PK phenomenon is happening at the post office because he works there. Since he is there, his aura is triggering my PK heavily in that specific environment, which is why this PK effect is manifesting there constantly. In other places it happens because I constantly trigger my PK, which affects the frequency of all telekinetic phenomenon. This kind of reasoning is important o analyze as aspiring PK practitioners.

I was raised in a small community in Southern California and had a good friend like a brother named Drew who lived a few houses down the street. He went into the military and we lost touch for more than ten years. He eventually moved to southern Mexico with his mother and I moved across the world for my studies. When I moved back from Holland into a very small city in the Pacific Northwest, I decided to perform a PK experiment one random day. For this experiment, I decided to carry my pendulum on myself for a full day and observe the mind over matter effects.

When I first left my home carrying the pendulum, I went to the small local supermarket. Interestingly enough, Drew was standing right outside waiting to greet me. We were both so happy to see each other agin for the first time in more than ten years! He said that he was only passing through for a short while, so we spent some time together for a few days. While driving around the city together, we both noticed that a large amount of cars around us had one front light that was not working. He was amazed at how many cars had this problem in around us.

I was discussing this "car light phenomenon" with a friend at a restaurant and it was the first time that we went out together. After I told her about it, she informed me that one of her back lights just recently stopped working. A few weeks after she told me this, I fortuitously encountered her again while walking through town. She then told me that when we parted that evening and she went back to her car, her light mysteriously came back on immediately. On another occasion, I was speaking to a disciple at his house about this car light phenomenon and how it happens so persistently. As we were walking to his house, we both observed a car drive past us that had one front light out. As soon as I left his house , the very first car that drove past me also had one front light that was not working. Of course, I told him how this happened and he was quite captivated.

By now, it is clear that the miraculous force creating the FP is not confined to affecting the electric functioning of refrigerators! The FP and other objective PK phenomenon are manifestations directly from God, which give our minds a direct structural connection to His divine omnipresent power. However, making this mental connection with the divine power is only the first step towards your spiritual liberation. In order to receive the full spiritual blessings from God, it is imperative that you believe in this Shakti power and openly receive it without relent.

One person asked me why God would not want people's car lights to work? My response is that we can never fully understand Him, but we do know that He will do whatever it takes to get our attention. Since we can not see God, it is often very difficult to make a mental connection with Him and have faith. However, we can make mental connections to His *manifestations*, which gives us a direct way of linking to Him. Since there is no difference between the Lord and His manifestations, these phenomenon are a structural link straight to God! That is the greatest gain in this human form of life.

The FP is God's manifestation of His divine power for this time and age. He has innumerable forms, representatives, names, incarnations (avatars), and manifestations. By connecting with these manifestations, the mind links straight to the power of God's hand. By merely coming into contact with this sublime power, our lives can never stay the same. The next two chapters enable you to study how the FP functions in greater depth, and to make an even deeper mental connection with this face of God. This automatically dovetails the mind with His omnipresent consciousness. The more our that our minds are connected to Him, the more our consciousness becomes like His on a quantitative level. This transcendental association gives us the greatest level of control over matter and brings the best fortune into our lives.

There is a well known relationship between PK and electricity, which is why many PK practitioners such as Alla Vinogradova choose not to do any experimentation during a thunderstorm. Scientists noticed a variety of interesting things related to electricity happening during her PK research. They noticed that electrical sparks were emitting from her hands, and that she was able to create an electromagnetic field around her. Personally, I love to work during thunderstorms and intensify the activity. I have consistently noticed this correlation between PK and electricity. On one occasion, I was chanting incessantly and very intensively all day. I went to turn on my light, and the light switch itself shocked me with blue electricity!

On other occasions I have caused lights to either black out momentarily or completely blow out during intensive chanting and meditation sessions with disciples. In psi research studies involving out of body experiences, it has been reported on numerous occasions that some have been glued to power lines after leaving their bodies. This shows some connection between our bioenergetic counterpart, the etheric/astral or pranic body and electricity. I have found that weather can also be extremely effected by the d use of psychotronics than run on electricity. Clearly God has designed material nature in such a way that electricity even functions on metaphysical and spiritual levels. All of these manifestations of PK are crucial for use to know about in this high-tech paradigm. In trying to use the power of PK to control our lives, we first need to know that it is real. They provide concrete evidence for me, all of the eye witnesses, and whoever else has the higher intelligence to believe and receive. All of these miracles are great blessings from God to teach us that mind over matter is real, and that we can use this principle to control our destiny.

In this day and age, we can not afford to ignore modern science in our "transcendental" studies. Our lives are so heavily influenced by its technologies and related advancements. Since the highest transcendental yogis commonly experience PK effects in their environments, we in the modern world should also expect to experience powerful PK phenomenon manifesting through technologies in our environments! This is the natural result of merging spirituality, metaphysics and technology in the new world. Moreover, since all of the breakthroughs in the fields of psi and PK research have involved advanced apparatus, we should focus on how technology can be used to enhance our understanding these mental forces.

In light of all the research confirming the existence of PK, it becomes apparent what force is causing this to happen with the refrigerator. In fact, my Austrian Guru who is a an expert in telekinetic technologies instantly recognized what it was. He is a biophysicists and an expert in metaphysics. The Austrian Guru was the first person who determined that my experiences certainly were distinct cases of True PK. Actually, without his divine influence in explaining all of it, I would be lost and confused about what in the world was going on.

The Lord Sri Krsna that spoke Srimad *Bhagavad-Gita* on the battle filed of Kuruksetra was by no means a passive or docile Personality. He also urged His disciple Arjuna to take action and did not approve of his decision to not fight. It is always the Lord's Karma to be active and supremely controlling and it was Arjuna's Karma to fight the battle so he did. The FP is a manifestation of the exact same active hand of God working in this day and time.   Ultimately, it is my Karma as a self realized soul that enables me to perform these kinds of feats.

By dovetailing the soul with the Supreme Soul through the practice of Bhakti-yoga, *anybody* can comprehend how theses things are possible and attain the highest levels of happiness in life. That happens when by recognizing that we are not these physical bodies and that our consciousness is not limited to them. The difference between God and man is that our consciousness is limited to occupying the external material body.   God's consciousness occupies everybody and everything at one time.   Krsna Consciousness results in our minds being elevated to the level of God. Since our soul is limited in power and the Supreme Consciousness (Lord Sri Krsna) is all pervasive, we can transcend the material concept of life by merging with His supreme soul. In other words, after linking our consciousness with the Supreme Lord, we too become transcendental, our minds and senses perceive everything on that level.

We change minds as we reincarnate but our true identity is pure spirit consciousness. That is the reasons why everything in existence is actually spiritual. What our minds witness and control is predicated by our level of consciousness. Our minds serve as pilots for the consciousness (a vessel) and obviously can control it. When we abolish the lower mindset of physical and bodily limitation, our consciousness does not assume a material body when we reincarnate. The FP and   other   paranormal   psychokinetic phenomenon naturally result from my consciousness naturally being elevated via dovetailing it with the Supreme.

In fact, the key to overcoming all miseries, distress and unhappiness permanently is to overcome the bodily concept of life. The various stages of samadhi that we explored earlier help us to transcend the bodily concept. That is fostered by practicing yoga. All of our spiritual problems are a product of false identification with the physical body and the material world. Originally, we are all Krsna conscious and somehow acute amnesia set in. This resulting from our contact with the material world and its particle. Those who have karma that is auspicious enough to see this truth and light are eligible for being situated back in the original position of God Consciousness.

Understanding that we are spiritual mobile centers of consciousness is the key to transcending all unhappiness resulting from material existence. By analogy, if one's physical body is afflicted with some problem and then the person dies, all of those specific bodily pains are gone. Similarly, when we abolish our spiritual illness of false identification with the material body, all of our spiritual issues such as unhappiness and misery gradually come to an end. This perspective also helps us to overcome material limitation and to naturally elevated the mind for optimum control over matter. The FP is only one manifestation of this, which removed the obstacles for us to perform crucial work for Lord Sri Krsna and His Vaishnava people.

By accepting my divine grace, the same cosmic energy that is manifesting through refrigerators all over will purify your mind, body and environment wherever you are. This same miraculous and divine PK force can make anything happen for you. If you want to be saved from whatever besets you, and surmount any obstacle with ease, then pray to Krsna, and worship Him as Jagannatha! You should then immediately feel the divine telekinetic force moving through your whole body. The Lord's secret *Sudarsana Cakra* disk will destroy every bit of your delusion, material inebriation, and false identification with the material world.

Consequently, your mind and consciousness will immediately be lifted to the highest levels of infinite power. This is the key to liberation, as the influence of *kali-yuga* requires the power of God's secret weapon. If you want to be fully protected and delivered from all perils, evil, and darkness of this age, then you had better worship Jagannatha with all of your heart. Again, in Srimad Bhagavatam, the most authoritative yogic scriptures, the Lord states plainly that we are to worship the gurus as His divine representatives. This is because there is no difference between Him and His most divine representatives. Of course, we all have varying levels of this PK energy within us. In the case of an avatar or representative of God, the quantitative levels of this energy are considered "superhuman" or "supernatural." Hence, people like us are able to perform certain feats that are impossible for the ordinary man.

Any reasonably thinking person knows when one thing is controlling another or is triggering it. That is exactly why I discovered the FP in the first instance, and why numerous eye witnesses have confirmed it. The FP is excellent as a concept for understanding how true mind over matter really works. It gives us a glimpse into the next level of human evolution. I readily acknowledge that some degree of telekinetic power can be acquired by anybody, through virtually any religious or spiritual path. So, I certainly encourage many readers to stay where you are in terms of your spirituality!

Krsna consciousness is not for everybody, but everybody can benefit from learning about the science of mind over matter from a our perspective. By merely learning more about the FP and true PK, you too will learn how to work with your own natural psychic abilities. Moreover, by merely reading this book, you experience an activation in your kundalini and PK powers. Of course, there will be many of you who are compelled to the highest road of transcendentalism and religion, which is factually *bhakti-yoga*. It is my personal belief based on the spotlessness and perfection of Vedic scripture that the highest degree of control and understanding of this cosmic force only is achieved as a direct result of *devotional service* unto Syamasundara (Krsna).

Rendering homage unto the Supreme Lord Vishnu, the Chief controller naturally affords the highest pleasures and powers imaginable. Evidently, I do recognize that amazing experiences with PK have been observed in nearly every spiritual tradition and religion. So you can also use my *experiences* as a template for developing your own understanding of PK based on your own personal spirituality or religious path. Of course, as an author who is also a practitioner of *Bhakti-yoga*, it is my karmic duty to give you the secrets of PK, while also helping you to understand the principles of true religion.

In terms of analysis and evaluation of PK force, the FP provides me with one of the easiest methods of understanding how it works. That naturally results from studying and observing this PK effect on my refrigerator constantly throughout every single day. When one has an intimate home-based connection with this kind of supernatural force, one can more easily understand how the energy operates on all levels. This is why I admonish you to take heed to my advice and use it for controlling your life and destiny. I certainly can choose to produce true- PK effects at any time, as I have learned to master the secrets through *Bhakti-yoga*, via psychological training and conventional scientific methodology. I have repeatedly tested my ability to do this with various refrigerators as you will see in the next chapter. My consistent mental control over refrigerators is just an idiosyncrasy based on my karma. Therefore, it may not be possible for other people to do.

God has given me the knowledge and ability to consciously control the FP, by releasing PK force from my body at will. I believe that this same force can also be used to influence everything in the outside objective world to some degree. In other words, I think that just as this force can be used to control a rather complex machine like a fridge, it can very effectively be used for influencing life as a whole. That is particularly significant for those of us who are seeking miraculously effective solutions for self-help, personal improvement, karmic restructuring and spiritual advancement. Everybody is seeking some spiritual truth or ultimate verity to rest their life on. Studying how the FP works provides us with a very concrete point of reference in spiritual science. This analysis is very compelling evidence for a semi-physical force that can indeed control the revelry of reality. The key is learning how to work with it.

In having a PK experience, it feels most exciting when it happens out of nowhere and Im not expecting it. On the other hand, when I exert too much effort to trigger the FP, it fosters mild fatigue, and physical pain particularly in the upper left part of my back due to stress. In many cases, I feel quite worn down for days after working hard at developing and understanding my PK in relation to the FP. One of my disciples came over for a yoga session, and he noticed that the FP was happening so strong that he insisted on taking notes about what happened!

During our Shakti energy session where we used my psychotronics apparatus, I saw his aura quite clearly. It appeared to me as a shimmering green energy field, and I am also able to see blue pulsating auras. I believe auras are a sign of divinity, elevated, intensified and amplified levels prana life force. In fact, when I visited my Sri Pranananda, his aura was intensively blue and pulsating to the point where I could see it all over the room. The FP proves that the mind can indeed control matter like a remote control. By analogy, the mind can send out some kind of a signal that can affect electric devices and technologies.

The 108 recorded instances of the FP in the next chapter also serve to help readers engage in deep introspection. That is one of the most crucial processes for spiritual realization. This self analysis and transcendental meditation naturally leads the soul back home to the supreme reality, by helping us to understand the true nature of everything. Although others may not be able to reproduce my exact telekinetic feats owing to the divine laws of karma, my intent is for this manuscript to teach people how to control, direct and amplify divine PK force at will.

By merely reading about my experiences with the FP, the mind is instantly pulled into transcendental frequencies that permanently vanquish lower existence. These experiences remove all obstacles, miseries and distress connected with material existence. As a self-realized representative of Lord Sri Krsna [Vishnu], it is my karma to deliver these exciting discoveries in the area of PK and mind over matter with the world; and particularly the FP discovery which I consider most noteworthy. This superhuman feat underscores the real functioning principle for all of life which is mind power.

Many prominent researchers maintain that under certain times and conditions, the human mind can take direct control over matter. I honestly believe that the FP is a standard for intelligence for this day and age. In other words, those who do not believe in the existence of the FP and accept is reality fall beneath the acceptable standard for higher intelligence and enlightenment in this new age. On the other hand, if one believes the FP and knows that it is real, then I think that person is to be taken seriously. The higher mind and the finer tissues of the brain can lead you to the absolute truth when they are awakened and the brow chakra is stimulated. That truth will set you free!

Chapter 9: Empirical Research with the FP

There have been extensive empirical reports of PK phenomena all throughout history in various cultures. The value of empirical research rests in the fact that it enables us to observe the object in a most naturalistic manner. One of the main advantages of presenting this kind of research is that it helps readers to understand the practices that are centrally involved with manifesting true PK and mind over matter. By integrating the yogic practices that I use into your everyday life, I believe that your mind's power and control over matter can be easily "carried over" into every field of life. That is the most powerful approach for self improvement, spiritual advancement and miracle working of all varieties.

Again, by studying these empirical records, your mind automatically makes a very strong connection with the hand of God in action. There I must reiterate that is very difficult for people to connect with God and put full faith in Him without observing His hand in action. Rather than imposing artificial controls on a situation, naturalistic observation helps us to see it all working in a more comprehensive way. It can lead to even more powerful discoveries. These extensive records are here to give readers a clear idea of how the FP works and how I perceive the discovery.

This medium of communication is the best way to delineate this very real psychokinetic phenomenon. I consider these records of my PK experiences quite priceless because it is hard to find recorded instances of how true PK works from the inside, where it relates to modern technology that we are all familiar with. That is only because true pk is the most rare manifestation of mind over matter. So many people have heard of PK or telekinesis, but they are not sure about exactly what it means and how it works. There are many rumors about moving objects with the mind, tipping tables, levitation and so much more, but what is the truth? As one who has first-hand experience with true PK, I have provided these records to illustrate how it really works in the most natural light. Since just about everybody has a refrigerator, it is easy to use it as a frame of reference for understanding how PK functions and what mind over matter really means.

1) I was sitting in silence doing some writing and contemplating the title of this book. I suddenly said aloud "This is PK," and instantly my refrigerator turned on. I thought it *might* have been a coincidence, but an hour or so later, I was washing dishes in total silence and randomly said again "This is PK." Again, my refrigerator turned on without any delay.

2) I was on the telephone speaking with Austrian Guru about my PK symptoms ones PK force. Within a few seconds after he began to describe the Telekinetic Wheel device to me over the phone, my fridge suddenly shut down. I told him what just happened. He was

amazed and suggested that merely describing this contraption created a mental connection that "triggered" my PK response.

3) I was sitting down in deep meditation and decided to do some pendulum dowsing. I could not immediately find my pendulum, but then I noticed that it was on my desk, so I reached over to grab it. As soon as I touched the pendulum, my fridge suddenly lost all power and shut down. After I was finished dowsing, I put the pendulum back down on the desk. Roughly one hour later I came back to confirm some answers that it gave me. Only a few seconds after I had the pendulum in my hand, the fridge shut down *again*.

4) I suddenly assumed a yogic hand mudra to metaphysically facilitate a situation I was trying to resolve "off the cuff." Within only two or three seconds after I assumed this mudra for spiritual power, my fridge turned on.

5) I was over my friends house and we were in the living room talking about the nature of the FP. I said to him "I can not totally control it at this point!" As soon as I said those few words, his fridge turned on instantly. At the same time it turned on a large leaf from his house plant suddenly fell to the ground. It was the only leaf that fell from the plant during our tine together. It fell at the exact same time as the fridge was apparently triggered to turn on.

6) It just began pouring snow here in town, shortly after I started carrying my stone pouch in my pocket. Snow here is quite rare, and I thought to myself, "It must be this pouch in my pocket." As I said that, I also put my hands in my pockets and touched the pouch. The fridge turned on as soon as my hand touched the stone pouch in my pocket. It felt like the stone pouch remotely controlled my refrigerator.

7) I stood right next to the refrigerator and did a small test. I assumed a sacred asana position. Within two to three seconds of me assuming this sacred asana, my fridge turned on. This time, I felt a strong magnetic force push against my body whole body as the fridge turned on. This was a rare time when I had the chance of actually feeling PK force.

8) After total silent transcendental meditation while at home, I randomly said to myself softly only these few words: "Nobody is perfect but God Himself." As soon as I uttered these few words, the fridge shut down instantly. This is something that I notice regularly, where I am silent for an extended period and as soon as I speak the refrigerator turns on instantly.

9) I was lying down in bed silently and totally still. I suddenly started chanting to practice a mystic mantra that I just learned for great fortune. As soon as I starting chanting the mantra, my fridge turned on instantly.

10) I performed a test with my psychotronic device, where I use it to project my PK energy onto my refrigerator. Remember that psychokinetic energy can be projected into a person or any object. As soon as I plugged the machine into the wall after setting it up to transfer the energy , my fridge started up immediately with no delay, just like it was jump started! On another occasion where I replicated this test my refrigerator shut down immediately and with no delay after I transferred the energy onto it with my PK amplifier. This small experiment has been replicated in my home many times and witnessed in household's of others including some of my disciples.

11) I was sitting at my computer typing for a long while with my leg crossed and I had been chanting for hours. I suddenly uncrossed my leg and as soon as I did my refrigerator turned on at the exact same second.

12) I was just doing some chores around my apartment and I started to chant as fast as possible. Although I may have sounded unintelligible, I noticed that after the third time I said the mantra really fast, my refrigerator turned off.

13) I was lying down in total silence and stillness. Suddenly, I began to chant and I already knew that it would most likely affect my refrigerator. Sure enough, as soon as I started to chant only one time,

my refrigerator lost all power and shut off.

14) I was chanting with my hands in the prayer mudra position first thing in the morning, Of course, I wondered if this would trigger the FP as soon as I began to chant! As soon as I stopped chanting and took my hands out of the prayer position, my refrigerator immediately turned on.

15) I walked up to the line in the local store, which was next to two refrigerators containing juice, milk, and food. As soon as I walked up to the line, I instantly noticed that one of the refrigerator units turned on as soon as I stood near it. Since the cashiers were quite slow, I walked out of the line to do some shopping on the other side of the store. When I walked back into the line and the same thing happened. Again, I heard one of the refrigerators turn on as soon as I approached it just to stand in line.

16) My Dutch Guru gave me a powerful mantra that I have always loved to chant. I was cleaning my home and suddenly I started to chant for the first time all day. Within a few seconds after I started to chant, I noticed that my fridge turned on. I kept chanting for long time nonstop. Then, when I randomly stopped chanting, I noticed that my fridge turned off immediately.

17) I was busy doing chores around my home, and suddenly turned off my psychotronics generator. At the very same second that I flipped the "psychic switch" and turned it off, I noticed that my fridge turned on.

18) I was lying down and suddenly began a chakra yoga process, where I visualize the sacred syllables AUM within my heart chakra. Within seconds after I began to meditate on these syllables, within my heart chakra, the fridge instantly turned on.

19) At a random time in the day, I turned on my psychotronics

device and started twisting dials. Within 3-5 seconds after I starting arbitrarily turning the dials that control PK, my fridge turned off.

20) One of my disciples was visiting me and I needed to get something out of the fridge. We both noticed that as soon as I touched the fridge door, it instantly turned on without delay.

21) Of course, another name for Lord Sri Krsna is "Vishnu", and one stormy morning I said a short prayer. I said only these few words. "Oh Lord Vishnu, O Lord Vishnu, O my sweet Lord Vishnu." As soon as I finished saying this, my fridge instantly lost all power and shut off. This particular morning was so windy that the sky in the city was filled with trash flying all over very high in the air like some tornado effect, and no one could control it. The winds were so strong that it was unbelievable and totally out of control. I think that this was a telekinetic effect because the night before, I was doing some heavy dowsing work and that is when I noticed that it was starting to rain very hard and the winds got extremely strong. Later on in the morning, I went to handle some laundry. I noticed that the soda vending machine turned on as soon as I entered into the laundry room. Then as I was leaving the room, I had a brief talk with the maintenance man who was holding a flashlight. He told me that half of the city just lost electricity during due to the whether and that he was handling power outages around the town.

22) I was lying down in total relaxation and silence. I suddenly sat up and at that same spilt second, my fridge turned on. This happens constantly and I call it motion over matter. This is a very typical phenomenon connected with my PK. Very often, when I am laying down or sitting, the fridge turns on as soon as I stand up, when I switch positions while laying down, or when I simply sit up after laying down.

23) I was writing down a psychotronics affirmation to use with my PK amplifying equipment. As soon as I wrote "I will for my PK" my fridge shut down. I had no chance to even complete the affirmation sentence I was writing before the fridge shut down.

24) On another occasion, I just finished writing down a lengthy

prayer to Lord Sri Krsna. At the end I wrote, "I will for my PK" As soon as I wrote the word "will" for the very first time in the entire affirmation, my fridge shut down instantly. This shows you how the element of will is the most crucial telekinetic trigger.

25) One thing that I love about Bhakti yoga is that one does not need to wait until the next life to experience the greatest karmic changes. Clearly, right here on earth, you can literally change your karma and witness everything improve right before your eyes. This is necessary spiritual advancement that reassures you that the spirit- soul will continue to elevate in your next life. I was sitting down and recited my favorite mantra involving name of Lord Caitanya only one time. I noticed that as soon as I stood up from my chair after chanting, my fridge shut down instantly.

For your insight, Lord Caitanya was one of the greatest and most influential saints that ever lived in modern times. It is said that He revolutionized the world more than any one else has in modern times. Much about him is unknown because he was very much shielded from the world by his closest devotees and disciples. The information about him being an incarnation Lord Sri Krsna Himself generally did not leave his small circle of disciples, who all knew perfectly well that he was an incarnation of God.

He is classified as an Avatar, and an incarnation of God Himself on this earth. As opposed to being an incarnation of one of the Lord's Plenary portions, Lord Caitanya was the proprietor of all Krsna's opulence as a direct manifestation of Him. He authored many wonderful treatises on transcendental yoga. Most notably, the *Caitanya Camrita*. This can be read, or downloaded along with many other excellent treatises on royal Bhakti yoga at the website: www.krishna.com. This treatise that he published is all about devotional service and how to execute Bhakti in the right way during *kali-yuga*, this present age of darkness and pervasive ignorance.

26)I was sitting up in a yoga posture on my couch in total silence, stillness and trance. I suddenly laid down, and as soon as I did the fridge immediately shut down at the same time. As you will see, many of these accounts involve me sitting or lying down, and then triggering the fridge by rising up. This is the exact opposite. As soon as I laid down the fridge instantly lost all power.

27) I was sitting down on my yoga mat, in total deep transcendental meditation, and as soon as I suddenly stood up, the fridge turned off.

28) As I was preparing a psychotronics experiment, I randomly set my mind machine to 20Hz. As soon as the dial reached the point of 20Hz while I was twisting it, my refrigerator turned on instantly. 20 Hz is the mind frequency for highly effective actions at a distance and for producing God's miracles using the machine.

29)I was in my kitchen and unwittingly leaned my back up against the fridge. It turned off no less than two seconds after I leaned my back up against it. The next day, I called my grandmother and while chatting, I told her how this happened the previous day with my refrigerator. As soon as I began explaining how I turned the fridge on by leaning up against it, the fridge turned on.

30) I just picked up my book on Kundalini Yoga, by Swami Muktananda. I noticed that as soon as I opened the book to begin reading, the fridge turned on instantly. Somehow the book easily triggered this psychic mind over matter effect.

31) I assumed the sacred asana position for powerful healing and within one second the fridge turned on.

32) I just randomly picked up my book entitled Krsna, The Supreme Personality of Godhead written by Srila Prabhupada, and I started reading it. Within only a few seconds after I began reading, I noticed that my fridge turned on. This is an excellent work produced by Srila Prabhupada, the founder if the International Society for Krishna Consciousness. This is a book describing the life and pastimes of Lord Sri Krishna. According to the laws of transcendental science,

there is no difference between Lord Krishna's name, His pastimes, his birth place, etc. It is said among the great sages that whoever has heard the pastimes of Lord Sri Krsna is immediately freed, and liberated from all material miseries. So, this book is a very powerful yogic tool that I endorse

33) I just started playing a sacred Vedic mantra. As soon as the song started playing on my computer, my fridge shuts down instantly. I noticed that this was happening very consistently ; that when I started playing the mantra, immediately my fridge was triggered to turn on or off. After a while of playing with this effect, I began experimenting with it and used it as a telekinetic trigger for my PK experiments covered later in this handbook. I discovered that this mantra was a direct way of controlling the FP through the telekinetic triggering principle.

34) I was getting emotionally worked up and it triggered the FP. When it happened the entire refrigerator unit trembled from the PK force, and at the same spilt second the FP happened, a car alarm was triggered outside.

35) I was speaking with one of my disciples in the local store where she works. She is quite familiar with the FP because we had discussed it many times. She lived in India for six months and was quite familiar with many of the yogic concepts that I presented. One afternoon, I was in the store and saw her so I went to strike up a conversation. As we were talking, I noticed that it was time for me to leave. Right before we stopped talking, I said to her " Do you remember that mystical fridge thing that I can do with my mind? Well, I learned to control it." As soon as I said this to her, we both heard a clicking noise and I looked to my left only to realize that I was standing next to a large electric refrigerator in the store that turned on as soon as I said " I learned to control it." We were both amazed and at first I wondered whether it turned on or if that was some other sound. She assured me that she also heard it turn on the very second after I told her that I can now control the FP.

36) I was reading the words of Lord Sri Krsna aloud from the *Bhagavad-Gita* to one of my disciples. I rarely ever actually read the *Gita* aloud, on this occasion I randomly recited this one verse, and as soon as I began reading, my fridge lost power and shut down. We were both mystified.

37) While reading a sacred text known as *Sri Isopanistad*, in total silence, I suddenly closed my eyes to meditate and uttered the one word, "Parusa." As soon as I said that one word it apparently triggered the fridge to shut down instantly. Parusa is one of the innumerable names for God, which means the "Supreme Enjoyer."

38) The time was 10:53 p.m. I spontaneously decided to run a small test on my refrigerator. I directly willed for my PK to shut it down immediately. Since I became aware that I am able to consciously will for my PK to do this, I performed the test. As soon as the clock turned to 10:54 p.m., my refrigerator shut down. That was only about 10-15 seconds from the time that I projected the PK signal over to the refrigerator.

39) I was sitting down silently relaxed at home in the kitchen, and I suddenly recited a sacred yogic poem. As soon as I stood up from my chair, my fridge turned on instantly.

40) I was chanting for a long time on my Japa Mala. I noticed that as soon as I began chanting, the fridge turned off. Also, as soon as I finished chanting at random it right turned back on!

41) I was meditating silently with a very clear mind thinking about how this FP happens so consistently, with such precision and intelligence. I suddenly thought to myself aloud and said: "I must be extremely telekinetic!" As soon as I said that one sentence, my fridge turned on instantly.

42) I was doing some work around my home in silence for a long time. Suddenly I realized that I had a bowl of prasad sitting on the

table. So, I took a break and went over to my kitchen table to eat it. I noticed that only a few seconds after I began eating the prasad, my refrigerator turned on.

43) I was doing some homework, suddenly stopped and decided to stare and meditate on a photo of Lord Sri Krsna above my kitchen sink. I focused intently on this photo for a few seconds without blinking or flinching. My fridge immediately lost all power and it turned off.

44) As I was reading about Dr. Bernard Grad's PK experiments with mice the most amazing PK affect happened in my home. As I was deeply studying his experiments, the fridge turned on and only remained on for 3-5 seconds and then suddenly lost all power and shut down. That is definitely anomalous for the functioning of any refrigerator. This was the same thing that happened during my own private PK experiments and testing. This is certainly one of the most interesting cases of the FP I have ever witnessed! There is a clear psychic connection between what happened to my refrigerator during my own private testing, and what happened while I was merely studying Dr. Grad's experiments. Somehow, by merely studying this experiment a telekinetic effect was produced through a mere mental connection.

During my experiments with the FP, the main thing that shocked me was how the fridge functioned in this exact same manner. It started up for only a few seconds during the experimental phase. Then it could not hold up to the PK pressure, so it lost all power and shut down in less than three seconds. At this point, the FP has only happened like this on two other occasions. The other time that it manifested like this I was chanting the Maha Mantra incessantly for a long time and completed more than eight rounds on my japa mala in one sitting. At one point while I was doing this intensive chanting in my meditation room, my fridge turned on, and then lost all power within three seconds. I immediately noticed that it was anomalous.

This is a clear indication that chanting is an objective scientific telekinetic trigger. It exemplifies how Vedic mantras are so powerful and have always been used effectively for mind over matter. What the greatest Gurus discovered in remote times is being confirmed here and now.

This also confirms one of my theories that the PK testing process and the apparatus used can trigger PK in a person all by itself. This principle holds true with all psychotronics apparatus as well, so by merely possessing such an machine, one can easily wield increased control over material nature for manifesting any desired purpose. This is exactly why this book is so valuable and so are similar works. By merely reading it, you become telekinetically enhanced and much more sensitive to the reality of this life-giving force.

45) I as watching a film on hypnosis techniques. As soon as I began playing the video demonstrations of the hypnosis, my refrigerator turned off.

46) I called friend of mine who is a monk that resides in British Columbia, Canada over the telephone. I could not help but to notice that at the same second as he answered the phone and said the words Hare Krsna, my fridge immediately turned on.

47) I was lying down on my bed with my eyes closed. I suddenly opened them and started reading a yantra script on the other end of the room that was written on a peace of paper. As I began staring at each of the symbols, my refrigerator turned on within a few seconds. Clearly, the script triggered this, and it was a prayer unto Lord Sri Krsna.

48) On one occasion, I was conversing with a friend over the phone, and she wanted to know where she could find a Hare Krsna Ashram in Chicago, Illinois. My refrigerator turned on just as I gave her the address to one of the Ashrams in her city. It was very interesting because I previously told her about the FP. She was amazed that it happened when I called her back and was giving her the address

during our brief discussion.

49) I began chanting on my Japa Mala and when I finished I randomly stood up. As soon as I stood up, my fridge immediately turned on, that very exact same spilt second. After learning more about how to control this phenomenon, I have grown to realize that the fridge reacts even by merely touching the Japa Mala or simply by picking it up.

50) As I was researching sacred yantras on the Internet, I suddenly opened up the photo containing a number of sacred yoga symbols. As soon as the photo appeared on my monitor, my fridge seized instantly, as it lost all power.

51) I was chanting for a long time in my kitchen while preparing some "prasad." After chanting the Holy Names, I began "oming" with special emphasis on the Grand Syllables AUM. I then needed to get something out of my refrigerator, so I touched the door to open it. I noticed that as soon as I touched the refrigerator, it instantly turned on as if I shocked it into motion. I was amazed and it sort of felt like when you mildly shock yourself after rubbing the feet on carpet.

52) I was drinking a cup of "charged water" with my arm rested on top of my fridge. I could not help but to notice that the same second that I suddenly lifted my arm off of the refrigerator, it shut down instantly.

53) After learning more by reading about my telekinetic potential, I was lying in bed for a while in deep meditation. I suddenly commanded that the fridge turn off by merely thinking the thought, " Fridge turn off right now!" As soon as I made this mental command, my fridge shut down instantly.

54) Lying down in total silence. At random, I suddenly whispered to myself two sacred words. As soon as I moved my lips to whisper

only these two words, the fridge shut down instantly. This is a very interesting form of the FP and it sometimes happens as soon as I move my lips and say anything after long periods of silence or as soon as I laugh after being totally silent.

55) I just began to read certain mystical mantras from *Sri Isopanistad*. Within several seconds after I began reciting these Mantras, my fridge turned on.

56) I was setting up a psychotronics operation on my computer, and as soon as I opened the photo (jpeg) for Sri Ganesha (The Elephant Faced God), my fridge instantly turned off.

57) While in my meditation room, I was totally still for a while and completely silent. I then lit a stick of incense, and at the very same moment I said a mystical name. Within 3 seconds, my fridge turned on. This is a great place to discuss the concept of telekinetic "triggers." Both the incense and the divine name are known as triggers, because they have the effect of instantly triggering PK effects. Other triggers I have tested for their PK powers are included later in this handbook.

58) I was lying down in total deep relaxation and trance. I was completely still and in a state of total ecstacy. Suddenly I remembered that I needed run an errand so at random, I rose up and only 1-2 seconds later, my fridge tuned right on.

59) I just opened the book by Paramahansa Yoganada entitled *The Autobiography of a Yogi*. I open began reading the chapter about "The Levitating Saint." As soon as I said his name aloud while merely trying to pronounce it properly, which is Bhaduri Mahasaya, my fridge turned on immediately.

60) I just began to hum a Vedic mantra and I was preparing to get a cup of milk from my fridge. As soon as I touched my fridge front

door to open it, I felt a strong magnetic push of the PK force at the same time I touch it. It immediately turned on as soon as I touched it. I stopped for a second and did not open it for a few minutes because I was amazed at how this energy works so intelligently and precisely.

61) I was in my meditation room and randomly started chanting for the first time in a while. I only chanted the Maha Mantra less than 3 times and my fridge shut down instantly.

62) While meditating in complete silence I said to myself these words," there is a superior form of energy making this fridge turn on, and that is what's causing this to happen!" As soon as I finished that sentence, my fridge instantly popped on instantly.

63) I was reading the chapter about the Maha Avatar named Babaji, who is known as the Immortal Yogi. While reading in total silence, I randomly said the Divine name aloud, "Babaji," and in an instant, my fridge turned on. I was amazed because it is believed among many powerful yogis that whoever utters the name "Babaji" with reverence instantly receives a spiritual blessing.

64) As soon as I walked in my front door after being away from home from a long while, I said the word "Krsna" only one time, and instantly my fridge shut off.

65) I was lying down on my bed chanting on my Japa Mala. As soon as I rose up from lying down the fridge turned on at the exact same split second.

66) I was sitting on my bed singing my favorite chant. As soon as I began singing I realized that my pendulum was lying down next to me on my bed, so I randomly picked it up. As soon as I picked the pendulum up, my fridge instantly shut down the exact same second.

67) One night I decided to perform an experiment by sleeping with my pendulum under the pillow. That very same night, this town had the most rare storm involving intense lightening and very loud

thunder. Lightening basically never happens here. The storm got very torrential and it actually woke me up. When I woke up I just saw lots of flashing blue light everywhere around my bedroom, kind of like a Polaroid camera. The day was totally clear before the storm and it was the very first thunder storm I had ever witnessed in this area.

I then remembered that my pendulum was under the pillow and that I was running this test for the first time ever! Then the lightening stopped for a several minutes and there was nothing but dead silence, stillness and darkness everywhere. I got up and turned on my psychotronics device. Within only a few seconds of turning it on, there was an enormous flash of blue lightening that brightened up the entire sky. At the exact same split second as it struck, my fridge turned on and so did my small electric heater, which randomly turns on and off. The lightening seemed to have triggered the fridge to turn on instantly with the heater. I have known among my friends in the neighborhood for being able to trigger lightening, apocalyptic thunder storms, torrential rain and abominable snow. This happened quite often during my psychotronic operations.

68) While me and a disciple were sitting in my meditation room, I randomly decided to teach him my favorite mantra. The split second after I began singing it, my fridge turned on and the light blinked in a very unusual way. This dazzled the both of us.

69) I was just leaving my home and as I was walking out of the door I started to chant. Just as I started to chant while leaving my apartment, the refrigerator turned immediately.

70) I was lying down in silence and meditation thinking about Shakti, its manifestations and incarnations. I suddenly said the single word "Laxmi," and as soon as I said this one divine name, my fridge turned on in an instant.

71) I just opened a website that had the crystal radio displayed. Within 10 seconds after I opened the photo and began reading about this old fashioned telekinetic device from the 1930's, my fridge

turned on.

72) I decided to review some information by Dr. Jan Pajak concerning advanced telekinetic devices on my desktop. As soon as this file opened on my computer screen, my refrigerator instantly shut down. Dr. Pajak is a New Zealand scientist that apparently has many telekinetic inventions in the works including a space craft that is powered by telekinetic energy. His information somehow acted as a trigger as soon as it appeared on my computer screen.

73) I was sitting down in silent meditating and I decided to begin some Oming the correct way (i.e. emphasizing the Grand Syllables AUM). I did two Om's while emphasizing this sound, and after my second Om, the fridge shut off suddenly. Then I stopped Oming for at least one hour and did some work around my home. As soon as I randomly sat back down at my computer and began Oming once again, my fridge turned back on instantly, as soon as I said it the first time.

As you can see, the transcendental power of the Om sound vibration is somehow triggering the refrigerator to react, which is a clear manifestation of mind over matter. Since we know that the FP is not limited to the refrigerator, it easy to understand why Oming has been used since the remotest of times for fostering a mind that is transcendental to matter as a whole   I always admonish my disciples to practice Oming properly for the greatest spiritual effect. This deep sound coming from the back of the throat has a strong purifying effect on ones entire being and specifically on the throat chakra.

74) I was in my meditation room having a sage meditation session while chanting Hare Krishna in solitude. After chanting nonstop for a few minutes, I assumed the prayer hand mudra and also bowed my head. The very next second after I assumed the prayer hand position and bowed my head to Lord Vishnu, my refrigerator instantly turned on.

75) On time I was in my meditation room and decided to clear my chakras using a magic bell. So I began at the crown chakra and rang

the bell while also chanting Hare Krishna and burning some sage. I rang the bell over each of my chakras and I noticed that as soon as I rang the bell over the last chakra in this meditation (the root chakra), my refrigerator instantly turned off.

76) My phone line was totally inactive in my home when I first moved in. During this period, my phone somehow rang that was plugged in to the wall, and I picked it up but there was no answer and just total silence. I then hung up totally baffled about how I got this call on an inactive telephone line. I could not help bu to notice that as soon as I hung it up and my phone headset touched the receiver, my fridge shut down at the very same second.

77) When an eye witness was in my home, my fridge was really sensitive to what I was doing, and he noticed that it was very much being controlled by my me. We were both in my meditation room and then we left to read a document at my computer about PK. The same second that we opened the file to begin reading , my fridge turned on and we were both taken by surprise.

78) I called this same eye witness the very next day over the phone and we agreed about how psychically wild and intense the previous night was. As soon as we stopped talking and I hung up from speaking with him, my fridge shut down and made a very loud crashing noise from power disruption. As soon as I hung up the phone from talking to him about the previous night, the refrigerator shut down so loudly that the whole thing trembled.

I then called him back and told him that the fridge shut down immediately after we hung up, and he agreed that it was very strange. He insisted that I make a note of it. This instance of the FP shows just how intelligent and real that this PK force is. It proves that whatever it is, this thing is watching us all of the time and controlling everything without question. That is what we are dealing with here. It is something to take very seriously and not to ignore any longer.

79) I was buying a soda from a softdrink from the vending machine in the laundry room where I reside. I began to chant in front of the machine and really wondered whether that would trigger it to turn on. It did not turn on and I was surprised! However, as soon as I went back upstairs into my apartment, the refrigerator turned on as soon as I walked in. As soon as I entered my apartment, I walked past my refrigerator and could not help but to notice that it turned on instantly.

80) I was sitting down at my kitchen table eating some prasad. Suddenly and out of nowhere at a random point, I decided to test my psi abilities on the refrigerator, so I mentally commanded it to shut down. Instantly after I sent the telepathic command to the refrigerator it lost all power with out delay. I shut down so hard and forcibly, that the entire unit shook. The unit is not old at all, and like so many other models, it is just very sensitive to my PK.

81) I was asked by one of my disciples at my home about a particular Vedic mantra, and as soon as I recited it for her, my fridge turned on.

82) I was laying down in silent meditation and suddenly began to touch each of my seven chakras. I touched each of the chakras for about one second. I began at the top crown chakra and then touched every one of them all the way down to the base of my spine. As soon as I ended this meditation, by touching the chakra at the base of my spine, the refrigerator instantly reacted by turning off.

83) I began my affirmation practices again for the very first time in a while. I said a particular affirmation three times and after the third time that I said it, my fridge instantly turned off.

84) I was siting down reading this book on Kundalini Yoga, and I suddenly placed the book down to assume a sacred asana. As soon as I did this asana, my fridge instantly reacted by turning off the exact same second as I assumed the posture.

85) I began my affirmation session first thing in the morning when I just woke up. This is the time when your unconscious mind is most responsive to your autosuggestions. I plugged in my psychotronics device to power the session, and I noticed that within a few seconds, my fridge turned on.

86) I was sitting on my bed meditating. randomly and suddenly I picked up a book on sacred yogic symbols. As soon as I picked up this book, my fridge instantly lost all power and shut off.

87) As I was getting ready to leave home, I noticed that my psychotronics machine was not turned on. I turned it on and also set it to "alpha mode," which triggers the corresponding brain waves. This was done to facilitate the day and foster consistent PK mind over matter effects for me throughout the day. With this kind of control over your life, every day is literally a miracle. As soon I turned on the machine, I started walking back out of the door. As soon as I walked out, I heard my fridge shut down quite hard and loudly causing the entire unit to shake.

88) On my way out of my home heading for the grocery store, I noticed that I forgot something and went back inside of my apartment. The same exact second that I opened the door and walked back inside, the fridge turned on instantly and I heard it turn on. When I returned from the store on this lovely sunny afternoon I started chanting and noticed that within one minute, it started raining. We were just talking at the market about how nice the day was. Then I turned on my heavy duty psychotronics device, and began worshipping Lord Vishnu with yogic asanas and mystical chants.

Within only one minute, there was a huge bolt of lightening and a crash of thunder that rocked this whole town. I kept chanting, while performing yogic asanas for worship unto Hari Krsna The Primaeval Lord. There was yet another enormous bolt of lightening that filled the entire sky with an amazing slow tracing streak of blue electricity. This telekinetic storm totally cleared up and the day got so nice out that I even went to the store and the storm was clearly over. One thing to keep in mind is that thunder and lightening here are extremely rare and uncommon in this place. Basically, they never even happen around here. In fact, the only times that I have witnessed them was during my intensive telekinetic triggering activities and experiments.

89) I began practicing a sacred *kriya* for the very first time. It is for producing good fortune . I could not help but notice that as soon as I started doing the movements for the *kriya*, the refrigerator immediately turned on.

90) I was lying down in a deep state of trance with my eyes closed. I was meditating deeply on Lord Sri Krsna as God Himself. At that moment, I felt and knew that He was God. Then all of a sudden, I decided to mentally chant the Maha Mantra. As soon as I chanted mentally only one time, my refrigerator immediately shut off. Actually, I was not surprised one bit because I intuitively knew that the FP would happen as soon as I decided to start chanting in my head and sure enough, I was right.

91) I was lying in bed next to my sage bundle I recently picked up from the local market. I decided just as a first time test to focus on it for meditation and see what happens. No less than five seconds after I began to stare at the sage bundle and intensively focus on it, my fridge turned on.

92) I was sitting down after eating a snack and then lit a stick of incense. My fridge shut down as soon as my flame touched the stick of Nag Champa incense. It was clearly triggered and this has happened many times in the presence of others who were quite amazed. This leads me to believe that Nag Champa incense can serve as a powerful telekinetic trigger. That is probably why it is the incense of choice within the Lord's temples. Once the energy is raised with a PK trigger, then the energy can be used to control matter. That is where psychotronics technologies come in handy.

However, it is also possible to use only the mind for controlling it, but in a technological age, psychotronics is definitely a prudent choice.

93) I experimented with a practice where I project affirmations upon my subconscious mind during the nighttime using psychotronics. Just before going to sleep is also when the subconscious mind is most sensitive to autosuggestion. This affirmation also included sacred yantras. The first night that I experimented with this, I wrote down the affirmation and the yantras, then placed it onto my heavy duty psychotronics device. I noticed that as soon as I turned my psychotronic machine on by flipping the "psychic switch," my fridge shut down instantly. What a powerful affirmation!

94) I was gone from my home for a while and the same exact second that I opened the door to enter into my apartment my fridge shut off. This has happened many times while I have been working with this energy in various ways. The refrigerator is somehow very sensitive to my energy field even coming anywhere near it. This form of the FP , which is triggered by my mere presence is happening in grocery stores and in the homes of others.

95) I was in the middle of an affirmation session right before bedtime. I was reading them from my affirmation book, which I encourage people to produce. As I was reading through them, I noticed that my psychotronics device was not plugged into the socket, so I stopped for a moment to plug it in. Only three seconds after I plugged the psychotronics machine into the wall, my fridge shut down..

96) I was lying down in bed with my light sound mind machine device lying beside me. The device is specifically designed to alter the brainwaves of the user for various purposes including psychic enhancement. This is the purpose of all "light sound" technologies.
I picked it up and looked at the front cover to select a mode for use. I noticed that within only a few seconds after I took the device in hand to select a frequency, my fridge turned on. It felt like pressing the

bottons on the frequency setter was a remote control for turning my fridge on! Then, only a few seconds later, I heard this very loud showering noise outside.

To my surprise, it suddenly began raining torrentially and quite intensively for only about one minute, then it seized totally. After about ten minutes, I got up and began to chant.. Then I noticed that my heavy duty psychotronics device was not turned on. So, I flipped the psychic switch on the machine and went on with my business. Within two minutes, as I was randomly looking out of my window, I noticed an enormous flash of reddish lightening right above my home. I was so shocked. Then, the hugest explosion of thunder crashed which sounded like a major bomb that actually shook the whole town from its core. Then it all seized and I stopped chanting.

Roughly one and two hours later, I just randomly started chanting once again, and I honestly wondered if it would make more lightening strike. Until I started chanting again, there was no lightening and I thought the storm was over. Sure enough, within a few seconds after I started chanting, I saw an enormous streak of lightening trace across the entire sky that came straight down from the heavens. Again, a powerful thunder explosion rocked our town, and then the storm seized. This is exactly what I call a very brief "telekinetic storm."

97) I was sitting down chanting nonstop for a long time. Finally, I decided to get up and do a yoga posture for raising the kundalini even more. So I got up and assumed this sacred kriya position on the floor of my living room. As soon as assumed the kriya yoga posture, my refrigerator turned on instantly.

98) I have occasionally been able to inadvertently cause cups to slide across tabletops by my PK. One day I was sitting down preparing to eat some Prasad. Immediately after I made the offering to Lord Sri Krishna, my cup moved at least five inches across the tabletop and then back to its staring position. So, I got very exciting and decided to trigger this movement intentionally. I used the Holy Names as a

PK trigger, and said "Hari Krishna" only two times. As soon as I said these divine names, the light in my kitchen blacked out for a full second, and my refrigerator instantly turned on. So although I was not able to make the cup move by my willpower, the attempt to do so obviously was unconsciously applied to the light and the refrigerator.

99) I was totally silent in my kitchen preparing some prasadam (sacred food) and suddenly began chanting. Instantly, the fridge turned on. After several seconds of it turning on, while I was still in my kitchen, I offered a bowl of food to Lord Sri Krsna and started eating. As soon as I began eating, the fridge shut down.

100) I was reading transcendental yogic and Vedic literature out loud for a while, which I rarely do because I usually read in silence. As soon as I stopped reading aloud, the fridge turned on immediately.

101) I was reading in my meditation room about some sacred mudras. Suddenly I assumed one of the hand positions and in less than three seconds my refrigerator lost all power and turned off. I then dropped the mudra and kept reading for a while. A little bit later, I randomly assumed another sacred mudra and to my surprise, my refrigerator instantly turned back on. When I left my meditation room, I looked at the clock on my computer and the time was precisely 5:55 p.m.

102) I was just preparing an affirmation and was not exactly sure how to draw the a yantra which governs will. I opened a file of the yantra's picture on my computer screen. As soon as the image appeared on my computer screen, the refrigerator instantly turned on like a switch.

103) I was typing at my computer for quite a while chanting the Holy Names Of the God. Suddenly I stood up and commanded my refrigerator to shut down by motioning my hand and telling it to "Go

off!" Within only two seconds, my refrigerator turned off.

104) I was curious about how my small psychotronics device functions, so I decided to unscrew it and open it up for analysis. I took the device in hand and started twisting off the first of the four small screws. I noticed that as soon I began twisting off the first screw, my refrigerator turned on.

105) I just woke up first thing in the morning and started chanting. Within one minute, I noticed that my fridge turned on. Then, I got tired and stopped chanting after only a few minutes. I went on about my business and only a few minutes later, I randomly started chanting again. As soon as I started chanting again, my fridge instantly shut off immediately.

106) I was in my kitchen and I my hip accidentally bumped against the refrigerator. I noticed that as soon as my hip touched the refrigerator, it instantly turned on, as if it was shocked into motion. For me, that was very direct proof for the FP.

107) I visited the library one evening and I noticed that as soon as I walked past the water fountain, it turned on immediately. I walked past it again much later and the same thing happened. I suspected it was due to my PK. As I left the library I immediately noticed a car across from me parked with one front light that was not working. Later on that night I had to do some laundry and when I walked into the laundry room past the soda vending machine, it turned on instantly. I did not want to be superstitious so I did not jump to any conclusions. However, when I went back down into the laundry room to place my clothes in the dryer, the same thing happened as soon as I walked past it for the second time. This totally confirmed that I am triggering this without question. Earlier on that day right after I was chanting I noticed one car with a front light out coming out of the post office just as I was looking out of my window. A few minutes later, just as I walked past the window again, I noticed another car with one headlight the was out pulling out of the same post office.

108) I was in my meditation room all alone at 1:45 am in the morning. Since I don't like running tests with the fridge using my PK due to stress, it had been a while since I made the conscious attempt. Again, I typically only make the attempt during my PK experiments in order to study the phenomenon. At any rate, while I was in the meditation room, I just happened to notice that the fridge was off. I suddenly and randomly decided to make the attempt to turn it on using my PK.

So anyhow, I willed for my PK to turn the refrigerator on. I boosted the test by using a special yogic mudra and a Vedic mantra to project the force onto the refrigerator. I then noticed that it was taking longer than I expected for the fridge to turn on. I chalked it up to a "psi miss!" As soon as "psi miss" thought crossed my mind , the fridge instantly turned on! I thought to myself "there it goes!" Then in no less than five seconds, the refrigerator suddenly lost all power and shut off.

That was when it dawned on me that PK was certainly responsible for causing this highly unusual functioning of the refrigerator during this random test. Earlier on that evening, as I was coming back from the local market, I noticed two cars with one headlight out at the same time (car light phenomenon). What happened is that I was leaving the market on my bike, I saw one of the cars to the right of me with one headlight out. Then as soon as I looked to the left, I saw another one with one headlight out and they were both driving towards me.

Chapter 10: Eye Witnesses Accounts:

As my PK experiences persisted every day of my life, naturally other in the objective world have been exposed to it. Their minds have been pulled into this stark realm of reality. Many of the eye witnesses to my PK have confirmed that paranormal activity is involved. This chapter is intended to help readers see things from the perceptive of an eye witness who observes true PK in action.

Case 1) While meditating with the Gita at His home, I definitely noticed that he had amazing mental control over his refrigerator. He produced a number of miracles with the fridge that I can not understand or explain. I almost felt hypnotized by what I witnessed. The most extraordinary thing was how he directly commanded the refrigerator to turn on and within only a few seconds it was up and running! While teaching me how to trigger my own "PK," he suddenly took a pendulum in hand that was lying next to us on the table. He waved it in front of our faces and in within a few seconds the refrigerator just shut off. That's when I told him that he was somehow creating a psychic "arch" between the refrigerator and his pendulum.

While in his meditation room, I noticed that certain words he spoke also effected the functioning of the fridge. For instance, he once randomly said the words "PK force" and instantly when he said those words the refrigerator to turn on! I definitely noticed that this paranormal functioning was connected to certain words he was saying. Later on as we sat in front of his refrigerator, he informed me that he had just mentally commanded the refrigerator to turn on. To my utter surprise, within less than five seconds after he told me this, the refrigerator started right up. Then I was even more bewildered. Finally, the guru took the pendulum in hand for a second time during our visit, and again waved in front of my face. Only a few seconds later, the fridge turned off.

Case 2) The Guru showed up at my house one afternoon looking for my roommate. No more then one minutes after he arrived my fridge suddenly shut down. We both remarked on how it was odd. My roommate was sleep all day long, so he stayed and spoke with me for a while. I offered him a cup of milk and when he touched the fridge to get it, the fridge instantly turned on as soon as his hand touched it! It was as if he transferred some energy into the fridge that shocked it into starting up.

Case 3) Gita told me about the FP several times and finally I witnessed it. I had not been over my friend's house for several months. Right when I arrived, they said that the Gita just asked about me, less than five minutes before I knocked at the door. He also rarely ever goes over to this house, so I know that coincidence or chance can not account for it. Several of us were in the living room, and as soon as he said the name Vishnu, the fridge turned on instant.. The light in the living room also lost power for a second.

Case 4) The Guru entered into my living room area and then we walked into the kitchen. As soon as we entered into the kitchen area my refrigerator suddenly shut off. Another time he came over and had a cup of water that he said he could use to make my fridge react. I did not believe him, but I watched just for entertainment. Within a few seconds minute after he held this water in hand and meditated, my refrigerator turned on. It was obviously triggered somehow by what he did with the cup of water. Another time he had a PK amplifier and used it to project energy onto my fridge. Within two minutes of projecting the energy, my fridge was up and running, and it was amazing to witness.

Case 5) I can honestly say that the refrigerator was doing some very strange things while I was in the Guru's home that evening. I said to him: " I have seen you hands, and you don't have any switches!" I was so amazed at what happened that I even suggested him to have a bunch of people come over to his place and witness this phenomenon! He then told me that it is not healthy nor good to do this for entertainment purposes, and that we should naturally flow with the energy, what it does, and where it wants to lead us. During our visit, we both agreed that this "fridge phenomenon" is connected with some energetic form of intelligence that can monitor us and even communicate with us at some level through that refrigerator.

Case 6) One night my friend and I went over to the Guru's apartment and spent some time with him in a meditation room. He said that he could make the fridge turn off with some energy field. He then lit a stick of nag champa incense. In less then ten seconds after he lit it, the fridge suddenly lost all power and turned off..We were all dazzled and quite amused. We laughed hysterically. While we all sat in amazement, my friend then asked Gita if he could also make the lights flicker. He immediately assured us that he could do it. He closed his eye, breathed deeply and within a few seconds, his light flickered quite noticeably, and his fridge instantly turned on! We are honestly impressed about how he can do all this.

Case 7) As soon as I entered into Guru Gita's apartment, my cell phone began to ring. When I answered the phone call and said "hello," we both noticed that his fridge turned on at the very same second that I said "hello." That same day, we were in his meditation room. He suddenly began to recite the Maha Mantra. As soon as he began chanting it, the fridge turned on and the light in the room lost all power for about a full second. I know that a power surge can make the light flicker at the same time as the fridge turns on. However, one day he was speaking to a group of friends in my room about bhakti yoga, and we all noticed that my light was flickering very badly the entire time, and it normally works just fine. I even told him that the light never flickers like that! This flickering light phenomenon is a separate "beast" altogether, but it it obviously works in conjunction with the FP.

Case 8) Within only a few seconds after I began a Reiki session with the Guru in my house, we both noticed that my refrigerator suddenly turned on. At first I thought it was a mere coincidence and naturally I resisted the reality of FP. However, the most convincing thing happened as we were finishing the session. Gita suddenly assumed a finger yoga mudra position. Less than two seconds after I saw his hand move into the mudra position, my fridge instantly shut down! I could actually feel the PK power as a magnetic push on my body! It felt more subtle than the air.

Case 9) One day as I was working at my store's cash register, the Guru came up to purchase some food. The total amount was $12.12 exactly, which immediately caught both of our attention, because the date was 12/12/2007! I remarked to him that it was strange how the total amount of his items equaled that day's date! Since then, he has come in and purchased items with the amount randomly totaling exactly $7.77, $6.66, and even $9.11. One of my colleagues named Chance asked him directly why this keeps happening! Another one of my colleagues also had a similar experience with him while working the cash register. We are all shocked at this persistent psychic phenomenon with our cash registers.

Case 10) The Guru was talking to a group of us about his paranormal experiences. He mentioned something about being able to affect the front lights on cars. Me and the Guru then drove over to a friend's house to see if he was at home. On the way there, we both saw a car that had one front light that was not working. I was quite amazed and told him how it was weird because we were just talking that phenomenon.

When we arrived at our friend's house, nobody was home, so we decided to find some other person to visit because we were so bored. While driving back to my house, Gita said that I will certainly see somebody that I know on the way home. I was totally shocked because only a few minutes after he said this, I saw my boss from work suddenly crossing the street.

Case 11) One day Guru Gita and I went out for some dinner. While driving to the restaurant, he showed me two cars, and both of them had one front head light that was not working. After seeing the second one, He told me that for some mysterious reason far more cars that usual around him have one front head light that does not work. While we were eating, there was another car right outside the restaurant with one front light that was not working! Still I considered it as coincidence and thought he might be crazy.

At first I was skeptical, but on the way back home from the restaurant, we saw at least five cars with front head light blown out within a very short distance. I was totally shocked. And don't doubt Him anymore. I have never observed that many cars with front headlights that are not working within such a short time and space. When we arrived at his home, I assured him that this only happens when I am around him and that I take this seriously. Naturally, I was very confused about how all of this is possible and what it means!

Case 12) I was sitting in my friend's bedroom with the Guru Gita and two others. We started talking about the flickering light phenomenon, and instances where Gita has done this at will. Immediately after he said that he can certainly make lights flicker, the light in the room totally blacked out for a few seconds! We were all taken by surprise and totally dumbstruck. After this happened, we all sat around in total silence, as we were speechless. Nobody was standing anywhere near the light switch and we were all sitting together. That was all the proof that I need that mind over matter is real. I have never experienced anything like that before.

Case 13) My mother and I went to the public library with my friend, and when my mom tried to leave, her car suddenly would not start. We had to push it over to another person's car who offered to give her a jump start. As we were pushing her car, Gita approached us on his bike while coming to the library. He asked us what was wrong with the car, and if it was an electrical issue. We assured him that it was electric, he wished us good luck and went into the library.

Roughly a half hour later, Gita came out of the library and approached us once again. This time, we were all standing in front of my car with the hood open. Again, he asked us if there was an electrical problem with my car! Apparently, he did not realize that we were the same group of people who were pushing the car before that he approached!

My mom reminded him that the last car he approached was her vehicle and that we were the same group that he spoke to earlier. Again, he wished us luck in starting it, and then told us that he believes "telekinesis" or "PK" is probably involved. Then out of nowhere, it started raining very heavily and torrentially. What I find interesting is that my car started right back up after Gita came and spoke with us about PK. I have a background in metaphysics and psychic matters. I think that our cars were somehow effected by some supernatural energy connected with this Guru named Gita.

Case 14) I have traveled to India for six months so I am quite familiar with Hinduism. This is why me and Gita have a special bond. He has taught me so much about spirituality that I will never forget. One of the most fascinating things that we have extensively discussed is his ability to affect the functioning of refrigerators. I was skeptical until I saw him do it for myself! On one occasion, I definately witnessed the FP while working at the supermarket.

We only spoke briefly as he was walking by. During this short talk, he suddenly said to me: "You know that fridge thing I was telling you about? Well, I have learned to control it!!" Immediately after he said this, the refrigerator unit right to the left of us made a clicking sound as it instantly turned on! He turned in utter astonishment and looked at the refrigerator unit. I confirmed that the unit turned on immediately after he said that he can "control it."

Case 15) I was standing outside with Gita when we were all of a sudden invited by my friend to come upstairs to his apartment. We went upstairs and in within a few seconds after we entered into the kitchen area, we all noticed that the fridge turned on. My friend and I openly admitted it was very strange because we had discussed it previously and I have always wanted to witness the FP. I had my doubts until this happened.

Case 16) While sitting at the table, I noticed that Guru Gita closed his eyes, while performing some kind of meditation. I suddenly noticed that my cell phone was on the opposite end of the table, so I asked my friend to hand it to me. As soon he slid my cell phone across the table to me, it rang as soon as my hand touched it. Gita noticed that the phone started to ring as soon as I touched it. He said that this telekinetic effect was caused by the chakra mediation that he was doing at the table. I also noticed it and thought it was uncanny, but I simply ignored it until he pointed it out. I told him that I don't think Chris Angel can do anything like that! I know this had something to do with the paranormal because there is no other explanation for how this can happen.

17) While visiting with the Guru in his meditation room, we began discussing his ability to make lights flicker. Suddenly while we were discussing this the light in the room flickered for a full second and his refrigerator turned on at the same time. What we found most fascinating was that at the very same second this happened, I got a telephone call on my cell phone. Later on that day when we were in his living room, I asked him for his spiritual name. At the very same second that he told me this name, the fridge turned on instantly! That was phenomenal.

Later on during our visit, he showed me a small mind over matter device that plugs into the wall. It was not plugged in but he held it in hand and claimed that he could remotely jump start his refrigerator or shut it down by using it. He then held the psychotronics device in hand and pointed it towards the refrigerator. Only one second after he pointed the device at the refrigerator, it turned on immediately. Just as he promised, he was indeed able to "jumpstart" the refrigerator by merely pointing the small device at it.

Chapter 11: Controlled Experiments with the FP

Based on the natural skepticism and criticism of others, and my own rational nature, I decided to conduct controlled experiments for proving the FP. I have known from the very start that the FP is a true psychokinetic effect. I have lived with it on a daily basis for nearly three years. Based on the way this energy functions so precisely in relation to me, it never has been a question in my mind that this is a true case of PK. These experiments are absolutely imperative for satisfying some of the skeptics and debunking the false claims against the reality of the FP and the reality of PK Force. My view is that any argument against the FP should be openly discredited and abandoned as an downright lie! I understand that it is a part of human nature to question new ideas, discoveries and breakthroughs. This proclivity in humans is nothing to be ashamed of, but we must not let it stifle our evolution. Instead we must use our critical nature as a stepping stone to success.

My friend insisted that there was a timer on the fridge. That had to be openly disproved, so, I decided to test his claims for myself, even though I knew from the start that they were totally false. However, this was the only way to confirm that there was no timer on the refrigerator. How did I know all along that there was no timer on the refrigerator? Because I knew full well that there can not be a timer on a refrigerator that is controlled by my mind so directly, consistently and precisely! Actually, there is no such thing as a timer on my refrigerator nor any of the others I have ever seen. Refrigerators do not run on timers. We conducted these research trials with to analyze the affects of PK force on my refrigerator's time cycles. The results of course like any other experiment enable us to draw certain conclusions about the nature of this phenomenon, and how it is controlled. Please note that the main purpose of our experimentation was to prove the validity of the FP and mind over matter "scientifically" using a unique approach.

Research hypothesis #1: The refrigerator's on-off cycles during the baseline or "control phase" of the experiment will remain quite consistent. This is the phase where only monitoring takes place, but no will-power/intent or other PK triggers are used to create any mind over matter effects with the refrigerator.

Research hypothesis #2: By consciously and intentionally introducing certain PK triggers into the experimental equation for the "experimental phase," there should be a significant and noticeable deviation in the refrigerator's on-off cycles. During the experimental phase, variables are introduced into previously controlled conditions, where the researcher only observed. The margin of difference between these two phases of any experiment is how researchers determine the effects of variables on the object being studied.

Theory: That the time cycles of refrigerators can be consistently, drastically, and markedly effected by conscious intent and will power. Based on more than 100 trials done to replicate these effects over the course of more than two years, we found consistent results.

During all FP experiments, the refrigerator door remained closed as an experimental control. For your technical information, the thermostat in refrigerators automatically responds to temperature changes and activates switches controlling the equipment. We started all trials by merely monitoring the on-off cycles during the control phase. Here we will discuss the results of our first experiment, where we experienced the most dramatic results. At first, the refrigerator stayed on for 10 minutes consistently. It remained on for 10 minutes, then it turned off and stayed off for another 10 minutes. We then continued to monitor these on-off cycles, and they remained consistent (10 minutes) for the first five cycles. In other words, for the first five times that the fridge turned on, it remained on for 10 minutes. For the first five times that it turned off, it remained off for ten minutes. I got really confused and wondered how in the world there could e a timer with all this PK happening?

During this very first trial, it certainly seemed to me that there was some kind of timer on the refrigerator causing such consistent on-off cycles! We used the clock on my computer to time these cycles rather than a stop watch. After the first five on-off cycles, we decided to introduce the first PK trigger into the equation (a Power Mantra) and observe how the fridge reacts to it. Again, we were only monitoring everything initially (during the control phase) and then we started using certain PK triggers (during the experimental stage) as variables to be manipulated in the experiment. The PK triggers introduced during the experimental phase are things that I have specifically observed to create a psychokinetic affect, such as pendulum practice, nag champa incense, and mantra yoga. This is discussed much deeper in the next chapter

Interestingly enough, as soon as I introduced the power mantra as the first variable introduced, both on and off time cycles immediately fell from a very consistent 10 minutes (5 cycles) all the way down to less than one minute. Then I knew I was on to something, so I continued applying other triggers (concentrating on my pendulum, holding japa mala, burning nag champa incense, and some yogic power mudras) and suddenly we both noticed something quite fascinating. My refrigerator was turning on and off at the exact same second as the electric clock on my computer screen switched times! In other words, during the experimental phase, I observed that perfect synchronicity was psychically established between the exact time when the fridge turned both on *and* off, with the exact second that my electric clock on my desktop computer changed times.

To delineate this even more clearly, when the clock on my computer seemed to control the functioning of the refrigerator. When the refrigerator turned off, the clock switched times at the exact same second. Also when it turned back on, the clock would switch times at that exact second. Without a timer of any kind on the refrigerator, it appears that some kind of highly intelligent force was at work causing this to happen. In the great words of Alexander Graham Bell, "what this force is I cannot say, all I know is that it exists." Here we are not using the telephone as a means of communicating with man. We are using the powers of higher mind and the strength of yoga for communicating with God directly. Apparently, the change in time on my computer was triggering the fridge to turn both on and off, as if the time controlled it. Somehow this clock on the computer worked as an additional experimental control during this first experiment. This synchronicity phenomenon between the clock and the fridge persisted for at least three on off cycles.

The major breakthrough in this line of psi research happened as we replicated the experiment. During the second trial, we noticed that in the experimental phase, my refrigerator turned on, and that it remained on for only 3 seconds, and then it suddenly lost all power and shut off. In other words, the refrigerator caught an electric charge and started up, and then it totally lost the charge and shut down after only 3 seconds of staying on. This is the most extreme variation in time cycles for any refrigerator that I have ever observed. It only happens during intense transcendental practices or PK experimentation. This highly abnormal functioning of the refrigerator only happens when PK triggers are being used extensively. In fact, the only other time that my refrigerator has functioned like that was when I was almost done chanting nearly ten "rounds" on my japa mala, which I basically never have time to do in one sitting. It was the first time that I had chanted that intensively, and the refrigerator reacted in the same way as it did during my PK trials. More about how to work with malas is provided in the next chapter on PK triggers.

After more than one hundred of these replicated PK experiments, we concluded that the case for the FP and mind over matter was unequivocally proven. After this drastic deviation in the time cycles during the second trial, the fridge stayed off for more than forty minutes, which itself is highly unusual. It must have been exhausted like I was. This proves again that the refrigerator was affected by my controlled PK. Refrigerators never function in such a haywire and haphazard way under ordinary conditions! However, one time I had disciple working with me at home in psychotronics research with the FP. The refrigerator began functioning in a highly paranormal way that was directly connected to me.

During this research, I directly commanded the refrigerator to shut off and in less then two seconds, it shut down. This is a feat that I have consistently produced with refrigerators. This disciple assured me that something very strange was going on with my refrigerator and he insisted on taking notes. He then wanted to check my hands for switches and asked me if my guru "put something in my brain" to cause this. Of course I had no contraptions or devices of any kind to cause this, because this is only true-PK--mind over matter. We are both educated and agreed that some kind of higher intelligence is monitoring us and using the refrigerator as a means of communicating. Perhaps this is a way of communicating with God.

It is apparent that the refrigerator functioned so irregularly during our experimentation, due to the psychic stress and pressure it was placed under, by my PK force. This reminded me of the striking results in the research with D.D. Home and the mahogany board discussed earlier. In both of our cases, nobody expected such phenomenal PK effects, but it was proven to exist out of nowhere. Now, we can prove it much easier using modern technology such as the refrigerator. The crucial thing for our intents and purposes is the mind over matter principle; and how this divine force can be controlled at will for self improvement, control over life itself and spiritual gain. That is the subject for the rest of this book.

I readily acknowledge that the on-off cycles for most refrigerators vary from time to time because there are no timers. However, it never happens so drastically under ordinary conditions. You can ask anybody who works with refrigerators or knows anything about how they work. This line of research has proved to me that the mind undeniably does directly control matter via the agency of certain subtle forces. We should never forget that the power of yoga and metaphysics as a whole is confirmed by rare phenomenon such as the FP. They are here to remind us that our spiritual work is not in vain and does actually affect the fabric of life itself. Even though many people claim to understand mind over matter and believe in it, they still have not been exposed to objective scientific proof that they can relate to until now. The FP provides the whole world with an entirely new perspective, standard and framework for internalizing the reality of mind over matter.

During my PK experiments, I unquestionably proved mind over matter. During the second trial in particular, we both witnessed a total breakdown in the on-off timing cycles of the refrigerator. The major advantage of this experiment is that it removes the obstacles of doubt regarding the mind's ability to interact with and control physical technologies including computers. Now that the proof of mind over matter and PK force is under control so well, and contained within a modern technology, we can *move on* with building new ideas and concepts.

I am aware that many people are overly concerned and even obsessed with having the ability to consciously control the energy one hundred percent of the time. Our ability to consciously control it one hundred percent of the time is always limited because our consciousness is finite. That is why only under certain times and conditions we are able to directly control matter, but God who is the supreme consciousness is always controlling everything and has the whole world in His Hands. We must seek to understand and optimize this energy which interacts so closely with the thoughts, for optimizing the brain's potential and power. As Albert Einstein indicated, most humans do not even consciously use ten percent of their brains! The real secret to opening up our fullest potential is to merely acknowledge that our unconscious mind automatically handles so much work on its own via our PK.

The unconscious mind is directly connected to the infinite intelligence and communicates with it like a radio. Our conscious mind can control our subconscious mind and influence the unconscious mind is conditioned for power over material nature, that is communicated to the infinite intelligence, which gives us this kind of mind power. This is why I notice the most phenomenal PK effects when I am not looking for them or trying to produce specific feats, and while also engaged in yogic practice such as chanting. Even the FP happens with much more intensity and frequency when I am not trying to make it happen. That shows us how the infinite intelligence makes it happen on its own. It can control everything else in our lives just like that refrigerator. You will read more about how the subconscious works in harmony with the conscious mind in the next chapter.

Chapter 12: PK Triggers

Mind over matter does not work the way that most people think. It is a profound science that the principles of *Mahayana Buddhism* really help us to understand. A rather obnoxious person once asked me, "If you can make thunder storms and control matter, than make a lightening bolt strike right now!" I kindly informed him that mind over matter does not work the way we want it to work or say that it should work. However, you should all note that I have been able to produce those affects at will. I have made lightening strike immediately by commanding it to happen! Mind over matter works according to God's yogic precepts

PK triggers are based on the idea that there are certain things such as words, symbols, archetypes, emotions, and much more that actually trigger the mind over matter effect (PK). Once awakened, this power can theoretically be controlled, and that is the basis for psychotronics which is covered in the next chapter. In yoga, there are certain movements (kriyas), mantras, mudras and yantras that have been long used for triggering specific mind over matter responses. Phenomenon such as the FP enable the PK effect to be directly observed, so how it is activated can be more easily determined. Psychotronic technologies are very sophisticated apparatus composed of integrated telekinetic triggers, which amplify anybody's telekinetic powers. Many items for boosting PK can also be found in nature.

Everything has scientific functioning principles and it is our job to learn them. We do not create the divine law. It is our duty to figure it out and work within its scope. We must figure out the scheme that God created and to work within that. For example, a man by the name of Dr. Edward Bach made some remarkable mind over matter discoveries pursuant to his karma. Like any discovery, his were initially observed in his private subjective world. Then they were found to control the objective world that everybody else is exposed to. The principles of Mahayana Buddhism confirm that this is the natural process, and the key is to control it. If one person discovers something valid in their own subjective world, then it is naturally effective in the physical objective world.

If the subjective discovery is valid, and not fabricated in one's subjective world, it is indeed valid in the objective world. Take

Einstein as an example. He made remarkable discoveries in quantum physics that many people never took seriously. Einstein's discoveries were only a product of his karma in his subjective world. So many people regarded him as "crazy" or "deluded," as they could not understand him. However, they failed to recognize the ancient principles of Mahayna Buddhism; That there is no difference between subjective and objective worlds, it is the infallible law of the universe. My discoveries involving telekinetic triggers work on the same functioning principles as all other discoveries and the key is to control it.

Bach found that certain flower and herbal extracts somehow trigger specific mind over matter effects connected to holistic healing. These breakthroughs initially happened in his private subjective world. Many people throughout history such as Nostrdomis have been known for entering into altered states of consciousness for receiving revelations and discoveries. In countless cases, these discoveries have been tested in the objective world only to find that they are indeed valid. Bach's discoveries have been tested by many in the objective world, who have confirmed the effectiveness of his remedies as a science. Others have discovered that certain crystals are designed to trigger specific mind over matter affects connected with the chakras.

In any case, a person who makes a discovery must first run a test to determine whether their subjective phenomenon or discovery is reflected on the objective plane. As you have seen, my private subjective experiments involved the use of certain PK triggers that I discovered in my subjective world. I have been totally shocked and amazed at the results of my experiments, where it all has been objectively substantiated. There are also ways of triggering the FP that I have discovered which are totally of a psychological nature. This is a great example of how we know that everything is really mental know that everything is really mental and why the mind alone can control matter.

Anything that can be consciously triggered is by definition under some degree of control. As one who has worked with psychokinetic phenomenon on a daily basis, I naturally have discovered a lot about how to trigger it, control it, and amplify it. I believe that one key to happiness and control over matter is to integrate these triggers into our daily lives.   In this chapter you will find a sample of things that I have discovered actually triggers PK in an instant. This is very crucial because these tools trigger the mind over matter effect which can be used for our immediate self help, personal improvement, achievement, and spiritual liberation. Most people are aware of these metaphysical tools ,but until now they had no clue at all about how they are related to working with PK and actually triggering mind over matter!   The major advantage of these metaphysical tools over others is that they are easy to apply to your life at any time, while they produce the most powerful and effective results. Other approaches can be very cumbersome and much too time consuming. They are often too complicated for most people to understand let alone integrate into their lives.

A PK trigger is by definition "anything that is engaged with the specific intent of triggering PK, and that has been confirmed to function in this way." Categorically, they are either of a physical or psychological nature, both tangible and intangible. This is by no means an exhaustive list of all of the PK triggers in existence. Of course, throughout your PK practice, you will inevitably stumble upon others that you find useful. Since traditional Western science has fallen into the trap of eliminating transcendentalism from the equation, I believe that they are far behind in terms of really understanding PK. This is why you should seek the guidance of a bonafide Guru who has mastered the energy and the secrets for controlling it.

In this chapter you will read about the tools that anybody can use to automatically create a boost in their natural telekinetic abilities. The key is to scientifically master the use and integration of powerful PK triggers, for exponentially amplifying your psychic abilities at will and on call. You need to run your own subjective tests, as there is no difference between your subjective findings and the objective world! This approach to living will eventually lead you to the plane of nirvana and oneness with the Divine by illuminating all of your delusion and material miseries.

There is a world of benefit for one who knows the rules for objectively raising this distinct subtle force to control matter. With adequate levels of PK energy, anybody can just about count their eggs before they have hatched. I know this to be true based on personal experimentation and experience. The key thing to focus on is the miraculous nature of the FP, true PK, and that we know what energy is involved. If we can "call it up" by using certain tools, then we can certainly use the same intelligent force for manifesting all of our hopes and dreams. It's a fact. The most authoritative yogic scriptures confirm that this energy can be triggered and activated in anybody. I have indeed discovered that PK can be triggered, and that is the specific subject of this chapter. If you want to control PK and mind over matter on call and at will, then you must learn how to trigger it! In a time where everybody is seeking effective solutions to their issues and problems, it is more necessary then ever to utilize this divine force for self help.

I know that sometimes things are so difficult in life that only a miracle can work it out. That is when you need a direct connection with divine Shakti energy, the cosmic universal force. Engage it for any purpose and watch the miracles unfold right before your eyes. If you know how to work with your PK, then you can witness everything function just like what it is--only an illusion. J.B. Rhine and a whole line of scientists that followed his lead have confirmed that PK is a very real force. However, none of them have made the breakthrough of how it can be considerably amplified or triggered. That is only because their karma did not allow for the manifestations that would lead them to know about the concept of triggering PK. While raising PK force is quite easy, the more difficult task is knowing specifically how to use and control it. Here, you are given practical, fun and highly effective ways of raising your PK levels immediately!

After you learn to "call up" and "summon" your PK with triggers and sacred celestial technologies, you will naturally adapt and learn to use it for any purpose. This is similar to learning the skill involved in riding a bike, playing any new instrument, driving a car with a manual transmission or any other skill. Practice makes perfect, knowledge is power, and the key to success is knowing perfectly well that PK mind force is unquestionably real, and not to ever doubt that. Doubt is the number one enemy because it is based on the lie that belief in PK is some form of delusion. By learning to use your PK for controlling "maya," this great illusion, any positive permanent changes can happen in your life. By triggering a boost in your PK levels you automatically begin using more of your brain's potential.

Like many technologies, the brain itself responds to energies which affect its potential and power in one way or another. Some energies have adverse affects on the brain, while others clearly have the effect of enabling us to use more of it. For example, excessive exposure to certain energy has proven to be potentially carcinogenic. One the other hand, exposure to higher levels of prana energy and other vital life forces enables the brain to function on levels higher than usual. This is partly because prana energy itself is a powerful trigger of PK, which empowers the brain to function on a higher level. It is helpful to know when you are using a PK trigger, so that you can wait for the impact.

With the right PK triggers used and integrated properly while amplified with modern psychotronic advancements, one can theoretically produce any miracle. The miracles that one will produce is contingent on one's karma. And, your karma can be changed through the practice of yoga, so there is no excuse for not markedly improving in this life. The key is to notice your karmic strengths and then leverage them to create anything you so desire using PK. Since the following methods involve different approaches for mastering the use of subtle mental forces and "divine power," they all technically fall within the purview of Shakti Yoga. PK triggers include, but are certainly not limited to these. By incorporating these metaphysical tools into your life, you will naturally notice that you have much more control over the whole thing! You should also experience an increase in miracles and telekinetic phenomenon of all sorts.

1) The Japa Mala and chanting mystical mantras (Japa):

A Japa Mala is used for chanting, which is a sacrificial form of worship. The mala alone is one of the most powerful telekinetic triggers. So, by wearing it, touching it, or making any mental connection with the mala, one instantly activates PK effects. There are usually 108 beads which is a transcendental number connected directly to the pastimes between Lord Krsna, the gopis (cow herd girls who worshiped Him) and His cattle. Buddhist malas also have 108 beads, which reflects how Buddhism was born directly out of Vedic religion and Hinduism. A mantra is supposed to be chanted on each bead individually, and then you proceed to the next bead in the same manner. One of the main reasons why Krsna blesses us so much when we chant is because it is a perfect sacrifice. God always reciprocates us and mystic telekinetic power is nothing to take for granted as a gift from Him. By making this sacrifice, one becomes spiritually purified. The divine kundalini begins to rise and telekinesis is definitely triggered.

Mantra literally means " mind projection." It is a powerful technique for mind control. Mantras naturally elevate the consciousness to a higher spiritual frequency. Every thought and feeling we have is associated with a frequency or "vibration." All matter vibrates at a certain rat. Our thought vibrations resonate with and attract similar vibrations. That is the basis for the Law of Attraction. Energy that vibrates on higher levels is associated with the spiritual or transcendental plane and the divine.

Through mantra yoga (Japa), the sound frequency of the individual soul merges and resonates with the frequency of that mantra or the deity that it represents. It is one of the most effective ways of triggering PK. In fact, my first experiences with the most powerful PK phenomenon including the FP were produced with these mystical incantations. Mantra yoga is an indispensable aspect of transcendental yogic practice. The Vedic records supply plenty of information about how mantras have been used throughout recorded history. There is an exciting story involving the power of mantra from Srimad Bhagavatam in the next chapter on psychotronics . It is clear that these sound frequencies can tune anybody in to the highest mystical powers and mind over matter potential. These sacred sounds stimulate chakra centers that correspond to the frequency of their vibration.

2) Meditation on photos or statutes of divine deities:

A classic example of this is concentration on the four limbs of Lord Vishnu, which is known as "rotational meditation." This is a distinct form of transcendental meditation (TM). Many of you are unclear about what TM really means. It is specifically intended to "loosen the slack" between the mind and matter, so that the mind can assume its transcendental positioning and power. Now you know that meditation divine deities are the highest forms of TM and most powerful PK triggers. That is true TM that instantly creates a psychokinetic reaction in anybody.

The best way to perform this kind of transcendental meditation is in a Holy Temple (ashram) where the deities have been installed. There is no difference between the ashrams and the spiritual world itself. That is why they are regarded as embassies of the spiritual world. These transcendental environments are filled with divine architecture. This sacred geometry has been associated with divine power since the remotest of times. While there are many deities that can be worshiped such as Ganesha and Shiva, it is my opinion that worship of Lord Sri Krishna (Vishnu) is the highest that we can go. It is also my view that worshipping other deities such as demigods has a potentially adverse affect on our lives and Karma. According to the Bhagavad-Gita, we should only worship Lord Sri Krsna, which automatically addresses all of our needs and leads to utter perfection in life. This perspective is echoed all throughout the Vedata in scriptures such as Srimad Bhagavatam. The more intelligent ones among us choose to at least acknowledge sacred yogic authority in our endeavors to cultivate mind over matter power.

3) Pendulum Practice or merely carrying one on your person.

For those who are unaware, now is a great time to learn about the power of pendulum practice or "dowsing." Pendulums are of two kinds: A rod used to find water and a piece of metal or another object suspended form a wire of some kind. The pendulum is used in divination, to obtain answers to unknown yes or no, true or false type questions. It is a powerful means of communicating with God and engaging higher consciousness.

While holding it in a suspended position, one can ask a question and a clockwise rotation indicates a yes, while the opposite rotation means no. Many great saints were known for their powerful dowsing skills such as Moses. As you have read, I discovered that the pendulum is a highly effective PK trigger. You can merely carry it on your person, or use it regularly to project telekinetic mind energy into the situation that you are using it for.

4) Meditation on sacred Vedic texts, such as the *Bhagavad-Gita* and *Srimad Bhagavatam*.

All Vedic literature and other transcendental information can powerfully activate your telekinetic energies. Although they are not supposed to be used for that purpose, this incidental effect can not be denied or ignored. This literature is of a superior energetic nature, which empowers the mind for controlling matter more effectively. The *Bhagavad-Gita* means "Song of God" and it was spoken directly from the mouth of Lord Sri Krsna when He incarnated on Earth as the eighth Avatar of Lord Vishnu 5,000 years ago. The term Vedic means "Absolute Truth," and these scriptures are considered the most authoritative in the world for ultimate spiritual verities. While it is not possible to explain everything about the inexhaustible world of transcendental yoga here, it is crucial for you to know its origins.

To direct the people in general towards the lotus feet of the Lord, Sri Krsna incarnated Himself as Srila Vyasadeva, for conveying his transcendental pastimes. Each of the avatars/incarnations of God have distinct purposes on Earth. In fact, there are different kinds of avatars. For example, Lord Ramachandra (Rama, "the perfect man")was Sri Krsna incarnated on Earth 2 million years ago. The spiritual epic known as the *Ramayana* illustrates His transcendental pastimes while in that form. The *Ramayana* is one of the world's oldest written artifacts and sacred yogic scriptures.

Srimad Bhagavatam confirms this in the first Canto, Chapter 3 Text 26:

"The incarnations of the Lord are innumerable, like rivulets flowing from inexhaustible sources of water."

According to Srila Jiva Gosvami, in accordance with authoritative scriptures on religion and yoga, Lord Krsna is the source of all other incarnations. He does not have any source of incarnation. In the Gita, Lord Sri Krsna explicitly says that there is no truth greater than or equal to Himself. While there are other incarnations who are called *Bhagavan* because their specific purposes, none of them are actually the Supreme Personality. Therefore, Lord Sri Krsna is known as "one without a second." He expands Himself into various parts, portions, and parcels all provided with innumerable energies, to accommodate the respective persons and personalities.

There is at least as much information concerning Lord Sri Krsna as there is about the entire country of India. That is why Krsna is the real spiritual gem and treasure of India. It is crucial to know that whoever reads the transcendental stories such as the ones provided in this chapter and the next about the incarnations of Lord Vishnu [Sri Krsna] is immediately freed from all miseries in life. That is the highest grade of transcendentalism and mind over matter. Merely studying the pastimes of these incarnations is one of the most powerful triggers for PK. On many occasions, just as I randomly begin reading about His pastimes, my refrigerator turns on almost immediately after I open the book or even touched it to pick it up!

That telekinetic effect is a sign of mind over matter power. It is the Apex of true yoga. Srimad Bhagavatam says that "the Lord is the inexhaustible source of all other incarnations which are not always mentioned." Srimad Bhagavatam also confirms that the incarnations who are not mentioned are " distinguished by specific extraordinary feats which are impossible to be performed by any living being.." So, it is not at all hard to identify a yogi that could be an incarnation, as we can perform specific feats involving true PK that nobody else can do. That is the general test to identify an incarnation of the Lord, directly and indirectly empowered."

Some of the incarnations are empowered with specific plenary portions of God's opulence. For example, Sri Narada was empowered with devotional service. Lord Siva was also an incarnation of a portion of the Lord's power. Maharaja Prthu is an empowered incarnation with executive function. Srila Prabhupada said, "the incarnations of the Lord are manifested all over the universe constantly, without cessation, as water flows constantly from waterfalls."

In the first Canto of Srimad Bhagavatam Chapter 3 Text 28 it states that "All of the above-mentioned incarnations are either plenary portions or portions of plenary potions of the Lord, but Lord Sri Krsna is the original Personality of Godhead. All of them appear on planets wherever there is a disturbance created by the atheists. The Lord incarnates to protect the theists." This verse distinguishes Lord Sri Krsna, the Personality of Godhead, from all other incarnations.

Avatar literally means "one who descends," as an incarnation of the divine. All of these incarnations of the Lord including Himself descend on different planets of the material world and also in different species of life to fulfill particular missions. Sometimes he descends Himself, and other times as His different plenary portions or parts of the plenary portions, or His differentiated portions directly or indirectly empowered by Him.

To further clarify this issue, Sri Prahlada Maharaja provides in one of his prayers:

" *My Lord, You manifest as many incarnations as there are species of life, namely the aquatics, the vegetables, the reptiles, the birds, the beasts, the men, the demigods, etc. Just for the maintenance of the faithful and the annihilation of the unfaithful. You advent Yourself in this way in accordance with the necessity of the different yugas. In Kali Yoga, You have incarnated garbed as a devotee.*"

5) Merely uttering divine names, such as any of the names of Lord Vishnu:

You will notice in the Maha Mantra for example that divine names are recited: *Hare Krishna Hare Krishna Krishna Krishna Hare Hare Hare Rama Hare Rama Rama Rama Hare Hare!* These Holy Names of God give us direct communication with Him. The more we recite these kinds of mantras, the stronger the bond becomes and the shorter the distance is between our consciousness, mind, soul and the deities whose names that we are chanting. Naturally, our goal should be to make a constant connection to the highest. Since Krsna Consciousness is as high as we can go, that should be the aim of all mantra yoga. While there are different spiritual perspectives it is clear to me that nobody can be more powerful than Lord Krsna. That is why we only should serve Him for the highest results in life. My discovery of the FP only happened as a direct result of chanting these Holy Names of God and worshipping only Lord Krsna. So I hope that you can see the supernatural results that "pure devotional service" can bring! By making such a connection with the highest power, we naturally wield the greatest and most remarkable control over the material particle and its energies. I have found that uttering certain divine names either while chanting or merely in reverence are the most powerful form of triggering PK in an instant!

A great example of this is the mere act of "Oming," with special emphasis on the Grand syllables "AUM:" In the *Baghavad-Gita*, Lord Krsna states specifically that He is "the Grand Syllable Om." It is the most sacred syllable in the Vedas. Unfortunately most people are unaware of the inherent connection between Lord Sri Krsna and the Om (AUM). As a transcendental vibration, the sound of Om gives us a chance to directly channel God's energies from the highest levels and tune in to divine power. This naturally results in increased control over material nature and a boost in mystical telekinetic powers. Whenever you think of Om you should remember that it represents none other than Lord Sri Krsna. It is His trademark!

6) Sage:

Sage is considered very sacred among Native American Indian tribes for one primary reason; it is a powerful trigger of psychokinetic effects. On countless occasions I have performed experiments where I enter into my meditation room and light the sage. Very consistently, I have noticed that just after it begins to burn, the refrigerator reacts by either turning on or off. It does not stop there. Other times I will merely pick it up and smell it, which also triggers the refrigerator to react in an instant. Many American Indians somehow picked up on its inherently paranormal powers, which I can personally confirm. Many of my experiences with sage have lead me to understand that it is very powerful for actually triggering PK if used properly. One can burn it, hold it in hand, smell it or merely give it an intense stare. Carrying the plant's vibration on your person is also effective for triggering a longer lasting psychokinetic response.

"Smudging" is a Native American Indian practice designed to purify and clear the bioenergetic field or pranic body. It involves burning many sacred substances such as sage or cedar wood. The smoke is then spread over the body and inhaled. I have been an active smudger ever since I was a young boy. The basis for smudging is that it gives the mind more control over everything by purifying the aura. Many Native American tribes also believe it is effective for driving away evil spirits, for good fortune, curing disease and other mind over matter effects. These substances somehow activate archetypes in the subconscious storehouse, which in turn trigger many positive telekinetic effects. From personal experience I can confirm that smudging is a very healthy practice that produces an instant and lost lasting boost in PK.

Saging is a powerful cleansing technique from the Native North American Tradition. Smudging evokes the sub-atomic energies of sacred plants to drive away negative energies and restore balance. It is the art of cleansing yourself and your environment using simple ritual and ceremony. For thousands of years smudging has been a part of Native American tradition but now its power of cleansing is available to everyone.

How can smudging be so powerful? The answer lies in the subatomic world of subtle or spiritual energy. In the Bhagavad-gita Lord Krsna specifically advises us that the spiritual energy is of a superior nature. Perhaps this explains why it can directly control refrigerators by triggering my PK. Homes and bodies are not just made of purely physical matter; they also vibrate with quiet, invisible energy. Smudging may seem a very modern practice. We read about city dwellers using it to sell their apartments or improve their business luck. But smudging has been used for thousands of years. When you light a smudge stick you are connecting with a spiritual tradition that originates from the depths of time.

I simply chant the Maha Mantra intensively as I do my smudging, asking the 'powers that be to remove all negativity and unwanted energies. It definitely works. When first doing this on a regular basis, you may find yourself feeling agitated or uneasy and not sure why. It is because you are 'clearing' with the help of the smudging. This would indicate that there is a lot of 'negative' energies in your environment. I do not have a set amount of times to smudge. You will find your own feel for how often for yourself.

Cleansing a space or our bodies with techniques such as smudging clears away the emotional and psychic 'energy debris' that tends to collect or hang onto us. It is a like spiritual spring cleaning. The effects of smudging can be surprisingly swift and dramatic. The rituals can help you banish stress, attract love, sooth you, or give you energy. I have noticed that it creates a powerful feeling of spiritual well-being. Certain fragrances are inherently associated with God and His transcendental powers. Nag Champa is one of them. By releasing this superior energy into the atmosphere around you, it enables your mind to wield increased control over the material energies. I have conducted many tests using Nag Champa and I have observed a phenomenal psychic connection created between the lighting of Nag Champa and the occurrence of the FP. As you have already read in the eye witness section, very often right after lighting the Nag, the fridge reacts

7) Pranayama exercises:

Hatha Yoga involves the control of respiration (pranayama). The term pranayama is derived from the word for breath, "prana," and the word for pause, "ayama." The basic purpose of pranayama is mental control over respiration with the object of slowing down the normal respiratory rhythm or even stopping it totally for long periods of time. Of course that alone can lead to altered states of consciousness that are certainly associated with PK. This is analogous to how the shaman triggers his PK, by affecting the brain itself through sacred substances.

According to principles of hatha yoga, rhythmic respiration serves to unify consciousness itself with breathing. Yogic breathing patterns are associated with different objectives such as health or for spiritual purposes. The act of breathing also supplies the fuel of consciousness. Breathing is a mechanism for accumulating the prana, which then releases the dormant energy kundalini. These breath control exercises are usually done in traditional yogic postures. The respiratory exercises are divided into three phases. The state of inhalation is called *Puraka*. The second phase of holding the breath is called *Kumbhaka*. This holding phases is followed by the exhalation phase called *Rechaka*.

It has been reported by some researchers that every inspiration of the breath is accompanied by marked electrical potential of the skin. This evidences how PK is being trigger by these exercised and we have already seen the relationship between PK and electricity. This can manifest as either an increase or a decrease in potential, in an order of about 10 millivolts D.C. Recall that Vinogradova actually had electric sparks emitting from her hands. Electricity is inseparably connected with magnetism and the life force. There is also a strong connection between PK and electricity as we have seen throughout this handbook. In fact, you will find that the most effective psychotronics apparatus and other mind over matter technologies use electricity.

These studies seem to indicate that every inspiration of the breath can be used to control the life force and for triggering PK. Without prana, the energy to sustain our physical bodies could not exist. When prana energy is recognized, cultivated, nurtured and enhanced our highest potential is achieved. Through harnessing prana and using other methods to control it, we naturally make the best use of this energy. As a result, tension leaves the body, the mind becomes calm and relaxed. In addition, PK is amplified which then leads us to greater insights and control over material nature.

When prana energy both inside and outside of the body is harnessed, controlled and optimized, it creates a boost in PK potential. For example, working with the"pranic body" to strengthen and boost its life force and the chakras naturally triggers PK. This shows you how the purpose of all yoga is not physical benefit, it is for developing greater mental and spiritual powers. While this may come as a surprise to many, at least you now understand why your physical yoga has also given you a far better standard of living across the board. Now you should take it to the highest levels and make

Bhakti-yoga the goal of life..

Pranayama techniques can either trigger or amplify telekinesis depending on the approach. It is extensively and traditionally recognized among both Eastern and Western traditions that each individual possesses a secondary non physical body. We refer to this as the pranic body in the schools of yoga. Under Western conceptions, it is referred to as the "kinesthetic body" and this image is encoded into the motor nucleus of the brain. This secondary body controls the breath and takes in prana, the life energy of the universe. When the pranic body is healthy, functional and working, one feels emotionally fearless and physically vitalized. Prana is the energy that animates all physical matter.

Most of us loose our prana constantly, which accounts for much of the complication in our daily lives. Through various yogic methods, we can hinder this loss and replace it. The more completely and consciously we breath, the more prana energy is taken into the body. We can facilitate the entrance of prana into our bodies, most easily through the top of the head. Sri Pranananda has a special method of pulling the energy in from the top of the head. For centuries, Eastern adepts have known that humans obtain most of their energy through the top of their head. Note that prana is energy is not PK energy, but rather a precursor to it.

Substantial levels of prana also enter the body through the spine and up the feet from the earth.. Perhaps this is why the kundalini is coiled up at the base of the spine, waiting to be triggered into motion by the incoming prana from the earth. As the prana energy enters into the body, it triggers kundalini into motion, which then moves through and stimulates the seven chakras.

The chakras are archetypes used to represent centers of physical and psychic energy. The major chakras are situated along the spinal column and are connected closely with the endocrine system. At optimum overall health, our chakras spin at very high speeds. Since they naturally slow down with age, it is crucial to maintain the chakras through various yoga exercises such as pranayama. This naturally triggers PK effects that can be controlled for any purpose.

8) A mere thought of something that triggers any strong emotional response:

Certain emotions have a direct effect on our subconscious mind, for better or for worse. God has designed man so that we are in complete control of over our destiny. I know this comes as a shock to many, because most have always viewed themselves as powerless and are not ready to accept the responsibility of being a demigod or "deva." Napolian Hill in his book entitled *Think and grow Rich* identified Seven Major positive emotions and seven major negative emotions. All of them act as stimuli that trigger an effect in the subconscious mind, which is directly communicated to the infinite intelligence. As a part of God, the infinite intelligence is all powerful and can make anything happen such as the FP! So the key to controlling and triggering this mind over matter effect in our lives is learning how to control these emotions. The seven major positive emotions are Faith, hope, love, sex, romance, desire, and enthusiasm. When we consciously integrate these positive emotions into out lives and avoid the negatives, we trigger our PK by positively communicating with God and inducing higher consciousness. This naturally creates the best of karma and good things arise out of this fertile positive soil in the mind. On the other hand there are the seven major negative emotions which include: Fear, hate, jealously, greed, anger, revenge and superstition. Bear in mind that there is a major difference between fact and superstition. When we entertain these emotions even unwittingly, it also stimulates the subconscious mind which directly communicates that energy like a radio to the infinite intelligence. Naturally, the infinite responds and projects that energy back at the persons's world which equates to "bad karma." This is also known as "reverse PK." As you can see once again, there is no difference between our objective and subjective worlds. Our minds control our destiny.

At some level, this form of triggering telekinesis and mind over matter is hardwired into the human genome. Major emotional reactions engage the higher mind or the subconscious. This can result in great mind control. Again, consider the elderly person who is emotionally compelled to lift the city bus off of her husband trapped underneath. This is a classic example of how PK can indeed be triggered by powerful emotions.

9) Metaphysical/spiritual paraphernalia:

Magicians of all times have used certain paraphernalia in their practices that activate archetypes in the subconscious mind. These work because they have been charged or "loaded" with psychic energy by others who has used them. For example, sacred pendents are direct *structural links* to whatever they represent. They are yantra archetypes which are very powerful in terms of channeling specific energies. By merely wearing then, you can also trigger telekinesis in your environment. It can be a powerful tool for mind over matter. After making a mental connection to the archetypes such as talismans, the energy follows the structural link to person. The natural reaction is the telekinetic boost because life energy is a natural trigger.

The ringing of bells is a long standing occult practice for one main reason. The sound somehow triggers a PK reaction in the subconscious mind. Many cultures have used bells in association with the banishing of unwanted energies or spirits. For example, this practice is quite common in the Russian Orthodox Church and among many Hindus. When used specifically for the purpose of triggering telekinesis or PK, magical bells can be quite powerful.

Certain stones and their combinations create a powerful force that can be used for general purposes. The effect can be so strong and remarkable that it needs to be discussed in relation to mind over matter and PK phenomenon. Of course, people from all over the world have witnessed the power of stones. They can be used to connect with certain chakras and frequencies. They are used for healing, general metaphysics, and many other purposes that involve mind over matter and telekinesis.

Many herbal concoctions from all over the world can be used as very effective triggers of PK. Herbs also can be used to connect with certain chakras and can activate them. The metaphysical properties of herbs are a result of how they can trigger specific PK reactions in the mind. Since herbs are organic, they are some of the most effective triggers of telekinetic power that one can use. That is why entire bodies of holistic medicine and science such as the Ayurveda have been used for centuries.

10) Using any professional "psychotronics" device:

Psychotronics devices effectively merge the latest advancements in the science of psi with the most sophisticated engineering capabilities. The purpose of these devices is to use a known form of energy (i.e. prana,) to create a boost in the telekinetic abilities. These devices can be very useful in amplifying and triggering PK, while helping you to control matter and the mind with ease. Many personal breakthroughs in understanding my own PK have been a result of using psychotronics technologies.

Psi researchers have established a connection between certain brain wave frequencies and the occurrence of ESP and PK phenomenon. These especially include alpha and beta waves, which are easily induced by using certain technologies including psychotronics and light sound devices. By using any of these devices for the purpose of fostering mind over matter and PK abilities, anybody can develop strong powers. There are many devices and machines that work on electromagnetic principles. They are designed to clear energy blockages in the pranic body.

Prana charged water is well known for inducing beneficial bioenergetic changes in the body. Some psychotronics devices actually are used to charge ordinary water with prana for overall health benefits. I have personally used many of these products to charge water and have found that they are quite powerful. I have noticed that for some reason after I charge the water, I am able to feel a major boost in my bioenergetic body as soon as it touches my lips!

11) Visualization techniques:

Visualization is to imagine, to evoke and to conceive. This form of meditation uses the imagination and feeling to evoke changes deep within the psyche and to give birth to a new state of consciousness. This altered state of consciousness is more often than not associated with enhanced mind over matter abilities, such as manifestation of that which is visualized. Naturally, visualization produces strong emotional and psychic responses that certainly boost PK abilities at some level. That is why visualization is one of the main tools used for self improvement and personal achievement. The best athletes use visualization techniques for success, but they fail to recognize that it is triggering PK that gives them a cutting edge over the competition.

Visualization is one of the most powerful tools in the worship of the real magician. Most TM practices and some kundalini exercises involve intense visualization. Thus, it is obvious that this invaluable technique has some connection with PK and that it can be consciously used to enhance it. Hypnosis is often a very powerful way of using the power of visualization to control the mind. Since hypnosis and other psychic treatment is related to inducing altered mind states, increased PK activity is a natural effect. PK is also triggered in the subconscious mind by various processes and often times hypnosis activates one or more of these. This is partially why hypnosis is so effective at changing the lives of the patients. Their lives simply can not be changed, without some effective mind over matter phenomenon.

12) Mudras (finger yoga):

Mudras are gestures made with the hands that direct and focus energy in particular ways. I have noticed on countless occasions that mudras directly trigger the FP. Many centuries ago, transcendental scientists devised ingenious mapping systems for the hands and associated reflexes. Each reflex is associated with different parts of the brain or the body. These reflexes are also structurally connected to emotions, chakras, physiological states and related behaviors. By analogy, foot reflexology is a classic example of how different parts of the body can be used as a mapping system for the whole. Mudras are used by yogis for triggering certain mind over matter effects. Some mudras represent protection, others represent love and others ward away evil spirits. In all cases, these sacred hand signs have been observed and effectively used for the purpose intended. Mudra yoga is a great science developed by bright transcendentalists and sages throughout history.

13) Applying tilak to various parts of the body, particularly when worn on the forehead

The tilak has a direct connection with transcendental energy, which gives it such phenomenal PK powers. In fact, it is specifically worn on the forehead and other parts of the body for the purpose of driving away "evil spirits." This is another way of saying that it enables our minds to control material forces, by somehow empowering us to vanquish all obstacles (evil spirits) in our path. These obstacles hinder us from living our lives to the fullest and certainly interfere with our happiness and spiritual well-being! Tilak is worn by women as a dot on the forehead, and wearing this mark has an immediately powerful telekinetic effect. Tilak is worn by the Vaishnava devotees of Lord Sri Krsna and also by Hindus. Although the Vaishnavas share this and many other similarities with Hindu culture, it is crucial to remember that Krsna Consciousness is not Hinduism. Among the Vaishnavas, this marking on the forehead symbolizes the heel of Lord Vishnu.

14) Sacred bodily postures and movements.

The ancient East Indian mystics knew perfectly well that certain bodily postures are connected to higher order energies. They also knew that these forces can be channeled by using theses sacred positions. These postures are known as asanas, and they are quite powerful for triggering PK. Asana is Sanskrit for "sitting posture," and they are intended to restore well-being, improve vitality and flexibility, and to promote the ability to remain in a one position for extended periods. Like mudras and mantras, there are countless asanas used for myriad purposes .By understanding that they activate PK through kundalini energy, we can take our mystical experiences and mind over matter powers to whole new level

The ancient Chinese Taoists were centrally concerned with health, vitality, and longevity. They believed that if they could live long enough, they could attain spiritual enlightenment. Their techniques fostered physical and spiritual strength and they are often referred to as immortals. Their methods include breath control, meditation, and dietary regulation. These exercises are effective at recharging the body's physical and pranic energy field. In this light, these exercises can strengthen and even trigger PK powers immensely. For example, Red Dragon Chi Kung consists of a series of exercises developed by adepts that benefit the body on all levels. It opens the energy meridians and massages the internal organs to keep them in healthy condition. This form of subtle energy work definitely benefits the chakras. It can act almost as a generator of PK force achieved through physical exercises. This is similar to sacred *krya-yoga* bodily movements.

15) The Ancient Gong:

For many centuries the gong has been used as a means of altering consciousness. This naturally results in a shift in brain wave patterns. Even scientific circles today recognize the inherent power of the gong for mental purposes. In yoga, the gong can effectively used for balance the chakras, to help eliminate disease in the body, and benefit the brains functioning. According to Yogi Bajan, "the gong is the only thing that can supercede and command the human mind." It is certainly an effective PK trigger also because it changes brain waves to the meditative states that researchers have already confirmed are associated with PK and ESP. So, the gong can enable us to take power over these supernatural abilities.

This particular drum is connected to the ancient and sacred trance. Again, rhythmic drumming is a powerful way of triggering PK almost instantly by altering the brain waves. The primary effect of rhythmic drumming on the brain waves have been long established by researchers. It is the basis of light-sound mind technology. The act of rhythmic drumming for extended periods in particular has been associated with altered mind states. These altered states are directly connected to PK effects and other psi phenomenon.

16) Affirmations:

The main reason why affirmations are so effective and powerful is because we are using the mind alone to manifest what is desired. This is discussed more extensively in the section concerning the telekinetic trigger of will power, which is the last trigger discussed in this chapter. Affirmations done properly trigger telekinetic effects by evoking throwing emotional and psychic energies into motion! I have found that they are extremely effective for mind over matter purposes. Some of the greatest men of the earth always kept this secret close to heart. Affirmations are positive statements that retrain the mind. They are well thought out statements charged with emotional energy. They must be repeated often to transform the consciousness. If done properly, the highly intelligent PK energy immediately begins to work on the aim of the affirmation.

Affirmations are basically a form of autosuggestion or self administered stimuli, which reach one's mind through the five senses. Auto-suggestion literally means "self suggestion." It is the liaison between the portion of the mind where conscious thought occurs and the unconscious mind itself. The thoughts that are permitted to dominate the conscious mind eventually reach the subconscious mind and influence it. This in turn controls everything that happens in our lives. It is very useful to integrate the seven positive emotions for triggering PK into your affirmations

Autosuggestion is a method of mind control, where the individual voluntarily feeds his unconscious mind with positive thought energy. If neglected and not performed, the principle of autosuggestion can work against anybody. Unregulated negative thoughts can easily pollute the domain of the unconscious. That part of the mind carries out commands that are well mixed with emotion. Many affirmations do not work because one fails to conjure up the necessary emotional energies and not triggering PK. Messages sent to the unconscious mind that are void of emotion have no effect on it whatsoever.

A good affirmation has five basic elements. 1) It is personal 2) Its is positive 3) It is present tense 4) Its visual 5) Its highly emotional. It must be visualized and felt. In affirmation, the feeling aspect is more powerful than the visualization. According to many leading researchers in athletics and business nearly every one of the world class athletes and peak performers are visualizers. The creative right side of the brain is one of the most powerful assets in affirmation work. Affirmation and visualization are mental programming techniques.

The most powerful form of affirmation that we can perform is the incessant chanting of God's Holy names in the Maha Mantra. When we do this, telekinesis is instantly triggered, while we are affirming that we wish to please Lord Sri Krsna. And when we please God, then all of the demigods shower down the greatest blessing upon our lives and environments. The Gita clearly states that all of the demigods are situated within Lord Krsna because He created all of them. As the Great Master Srila Prabhupada provides, when we please Krsna, there is no need to worship any of the other demigods because they are automatically appeased by our Bhakti devotional service. There are many ways of triggering telekinesis, PK or psi power, but I must advise that the most powerful trigger is perpetually worshipping the Supreme Personality of Godhead Hari. Krsna Consciousness is as high as you can go.

17) Cakra (Chakra) therapy:

Chakra therapy is a seriously powerful way of triggering PK and the mind over matter effect in specific areas of your life. There are myriad approaches to working with the chakras for conditioning and cleansing. There are seven major chakras. From top to bottom: The crown chakra is at the top of the head, the third eye chakra is between the brows, the throat chakra is situated on the throat, the heart chakra is between the chest in the heart region and the solar plexus chakra is in the solar plexus. The sacral chakra is two inches below the bellie and the root chakra lies at the base of the spine. These are sacred energy centers which each represent different areas of our lives and spirituality.

Each of the chakras is connected to so many different things that can be used to tune in to its frequency. For example, the solar plexus chakra is inherently connected to the sun. Therefore, solar meditation enables us to "log on" or "tune in" to the solar plexus chakra region and its specific powers. We then can operate from that plane, while triggering PK for particular purposes related to that chakra. In solar meditation, you sit in the sun and meditate on the name of Sri Krsna and His Syamasundara form, visualizing the light rays entering into your solar plexus. The light easily vanquishes all darkness and evil within us. This is certainly a great example of how to trigger PK through chakra therapy.

18) Feng Shui Practice

Feng Shui pertains to flow of Chi energy and how our environment affects its flow. Prana energy is known as "Chi" within Chinese culture. Often times while performing Feng Shui rearrangements in my home, the refrigerator reacts as soon as I start moving things around for better Feng Shui! For example, on one occasion, I noticed that there were a few items blocking my front doorway, which is not good for the chi flow. I could not help but to notice that my refrigerator turned on immediately after I began to clear out my doorway.

When I first began to practice Feng Shui, I just happened to remember that both bathroom doors and toilet lids should remain closed as much as possible. As soon as I made sure the toilet lid was closed and then closed my bathroom door, I glanced out of the window and immediately saw a car with one front light blown out! Of course, I could not help but to notice this amazing synchronicity. I was instantly astonished at how this Feng Shui involvement seemed to trigger my PK so quickly.

Moreover, within only a few seconds of seeing that car pass by with one light out, my refrigerator suddenly shut down and lost all power. The manner in which Feng Shui rearrangements have triggered the FP leads me to believe that it certainly is connected PK. Hence, Fung Shu as a science should be taken seriously. Until more recent times, the power of Feng Shui for mind over matter remained a well-guarded secret among elite rulers. Many great emperors and leaders from all around the world have been known for their interest and involvement with Feng Shui.

19) The Power of Will/ "Willing"

And last but not least, I theorize that one of the most powerful triggers of PK is Human will power! In fact, I have found in my work with mind over matter that it is the power of the will that is the key to manifestation! Since the good Lord has given us all free will, we are able to create as we please because it is the will that can move mountains in our lives. It's the will power that is at the center of disciplinary yoga which is the highest of all achievements in this life. The power of will not only triggers the power of PK, it also activates a lot of other psi powers such as ESP, telepathy, bi-location phenomenon, precognition, clairvoyance, and astral projection. The will is one of the four main pillars of the temple of King Solomon which are: 1) To know 2)to will 3) To dare 4) and to keep silent. The will has so much power simply because it is the mind and the brian itself, which has evolved over millions of years, that is responsible for mind over matter. As we will se in the next chapter, there are many technologies that radically boost the power of the mind known as "psychotronics."

However, we can not get confused into thinking that it is the technology that is doing the work. Its your mind that has the potential to control matter like a remote control, just as my mind is able to control refrigerators in this manner. Your mind is just like an independent energy field that is more subtle than matter and can easily control it.   Just run a few tests with the will power and the mind alone, then evaluate your results! I can guarantee that you will do it again because you will be amazed at the reults of directly your will power. Just use your mind to directly will for whatever you wish to create. Of course, your results will be drastically improved by using psychotronics in conjunction with the will and mind powers.

Its analogous to your physical body walking verses riding a bike, driving a car flying a plane or even a space shuttle! The physical body is doing the work via the person's will and the technology empowers the body to do things that are otherwise impossible. That is the best way of understanding how the mind machine works. Disciplinary yoga is ideal for strengthening one's will power because it takes great will power to control the senses! For example in Bhakti Yoga, one is supposed to refrain from all meat eating, intoxication of any kind, all elicit sex, and also no gambling of any form; and that includes investing in clearly risky businesses and academic endeavors. That is all a sacrifice unto Lord Sri Krsna, and Bhakti also involves that repetitious chanting of the Lord's Holy names which also requires great will power. In fact, I admonish all readers to engage in Bhakti Yoga as the best way of strengthen the will.

Give up those hamburgers and chicken wings. No more beer leading you into being drunk, no more casinos and no sleeping around! That's when the real magick starts in your life because you are wielding control over the entire realm of will. That is the highest yogic standard. If we want to create the lives that we have always wanted, we have to surrender the urges that we have to cheat others, or to trample upon them when they are in need. That is the only way we can create the world that we really want within the deepest recesses of our consciousness. The highest application of will power is using it to merge with the Supreme Lord in yoga. We must will for Sri Krsna to purify our hearts everyday by chanting the Maha mantra incessantly! Then positive permanent change will surely be produced in our lives.

In addition, the precepts from Mahayana Buddhism discussed earlier in this manual also empower us to understand our constitutional positions much better. Please note that these kinds of concepts are quite flexible and are not construed in mutually exclusive ways. They are to be interpreted and utilized in myriad ways. In that way they are quite useful for helping us to understand ultimate reality and the absolute truth regarding life itself. they are centrally important in terms of working with our will power. In life, we are all searching for the truth about its nature and verities. I believe that this concept from Mahayana Buddhism explored throughout this book helps us to understand the truth about mind over matter. Here, we are concerned with how this precept can be used to enhance the telekintic trigger of will power. We are also concerned with the existence of two worlds (objective and subjective) that can be sharply distinguished and used to perceive of reality in different ways. Our objective and subjective and worlds are analogous to "public" and "private" worlds respectively. We are all basically living in different worlds right here on this planet pursuant to our karmic difference. One person leads a life that is totally different than others, very similar to how no two foot prints or fingerprints are the same. We all interact with totally different people and experiences everyday within our own private worlds. Just as what happens in the dream state is typically irrelevant to what is going on in the walking state, what happens in one person's subjective world is not relevant to all others! That is why our individual worlds are regarded as subjective.

The truth about these subjective worlds is that they are controlled by our will power. Things that seem to be miraculous such as the FP discovery only prove that *literally anything can happen* in our own private subjective worlds. Moreover, the FP in particular shows us just how the element of will can directly make anything happen in our worlds. When we say that there is no difference between these two world, what it means in this analytical context is that the *private world* is no less valid than the *public world*. And, by opting to live entirely within ones own private world, one is liberated from all misery, as one is master of that world. So, this is one way for us to connect with enlightenment, by meditating on this Buddhistic precept that originated in the Vedas. Again, it is our natural right to create whatever we will in our objective worlds by using the mind alone, and we have the choice to live in that world alone. This requires one to tune the mind in to one's own private world instead of perpetually surrendering, conforming or subscribing to the public world , which is a frequency that is controlled by other influences. When the mind perpetually exists in this "public" frequency, it is not positioned to use the power of will effectively.

When we rely on to the public frequency that we have been conditioned into, it naturally leads to powerlessness. We are socialized to live and rely on the external/"public" world rather than focusing on and developing that subjective place, where we have totally different constitutional abilities and powers. Its all a matter of which frequency you choose to live on. For the sake of using will as a PK trigger, it is crucial to tune in to your own private and subjective world where nothing can fetter your creative powers. Since there is no difference between these two worlds in terms of their *validity and legitimacy*, the enlightened yogi decides to exist only in that world where he is literally a "god" and Master of Will. This is one of the best concepts for taking strong control over matter and life itself, mainly because it positions the yogi to understand mind over matter on the most profound levels. As soon as the yogi knows that all of her mystic powers and extreme control over material nature are only a natural result of her being the "goddess" of her own private and subjective world, then she is liberated and eligible for nirvana. Such mystical knowledge affects the mind in that way.

We all have control over our worlds as "gods" within them because we created them; and we are largely responsible for how they unfolded. When one's will is applied for manifesting something, then that which is manifested comes directly from one's mind. So, it follows that since it was born from one's mind, it is an intrinsic part of the mind. That is exactly why the great gurus, sages and mystics have espoused that "everything is mental," phantasmagoria and illusory. It is crucial to note that everything is one ane there is really no duality between mind and matter. They are both only energy and the Gita confirms that the mind of a higher grade of energy. That means mind can not only control matter in can throw matter into motion and literally give birth to material phenomenon. This accounts for why all of our most subtle thoughts, emotions and attitudes are reflected in the "external" physical world; and, it explains how there can be no difference between mental (subjective) and physical/material (subjective) worlds. It is all mind and largely controlled by the will.

Chapter 13: Psychotronic Apparatus

This chapter concerns how cutting edge psi technology can be effectively used to enhance our mind's ability to control matter and the revelry of reality. Due to its unbelievable complexity, it is not likely that anybody in parapsychology today can offer a comprehensive theory to explain how PK operates. Such a theory would need to account for all its different manifestation and the mechanics used to carry them out. PK is too complex of a mystery to be accounted for by neat rigid theories. When modern science does fully understand PK, it would probably take hundreds of pages just outline the physics behind its functioning principles. The first question we must ask is whether PK is a physical force or whether it is cosmic? There are two ways of looking at this.

Either PK uses or is some sort of material energy and biological force generated by the organism which mediates between mind and matter, or its manifestations are the product of a direct interaction between mind and matter. If the latter is true, we can discharge theories such as bioplasma, psychic fluid, psi energy, and psychic force. Actually, the research of many investigators already discussed indicates that PK is a measurable force that adheres to laws very different from those which govern physical forces and energies.

A few contemporary scientists are beginning to wonder if there is such a thing as psychic force at all. Dr. John Belhoff believes that this might be the most fruitful approach to the study of PK. In his 1975 address to the Society for Psychical Research, Dr. Beloff pointed out that physical science is guided by certain assumptions, principle among those that the world and all that transpires in it must be explainable by "impersonal forces." He indicates that PK may present a complicated factor and in particular:

"Under certain conditions, still to be established, an idea or intention in the mind can automatically constrain a physical system to act in such as way as to express the idea of intention. That this is in the last resort an ultimate fact about the world; there is no further bridging mechanism, to be invoked to make this fact intelligible."

In terms of psychic energy, Bloff has a has a very skeptical attitude about its existence. He said some theories like to explain psychic healing as due to a flow of psychic energy from the healer to the patient, a view incidentally that is encouraged by the healers themselves. Although many researchers in the West doubt the existence of a psychic energy, other scientists in Russia and India for example think that it is a central part of how PK works. In my view, it is clear that some psychic energy such as prana and kundalini are centrally involved with manifestations of mind over matter and psychokinesis. This view is also supported by the most authoritative scriptures on yoga and metaphysics.

Psychotronics is a term that describes the merging of psi advancements and engineering technology. It is literally "the projection or transmission of mental energy by an individual or collective metal discipline or control, or by an energy emitting device." It is also regarded as projection of mental energy so amplified that it actually becomes a physical or chemical force. According to many researchers, scientists in some nations have made significant progress towards practical application of PK energy.

It has been argued by many US government officers that it is possible to use this energy as a significant military force. However, due to the secrecy of weaponry development, it is hard to know how far along PK weaponry development is. For our intents and purposes, we are of course only concerned with how these technologies can be used to enhance our lives for self-improvement and spiritual advancement. On the other hand, it is always interesting to observe how psychotronics energies have been utilized throughout history.

Based on the results of many research studies including some conducted with Indigo Swann at the Stanford Research Institute, the US government considered the possibility psychic warfare a serious international issue. In response to the growing international threats involved with psychic warfare, many US government officials and agencies admonish the whole world to remain open minded about PK developments. In 1981 the authors of a partly declassified U.S. Army report emphasized the importance of "remaining open-minded about psychokinesis." They consider PK as a form of energy with "potentially serious military applications."

In this same report the military officials reported that some countries have "made significant progress toward developing psychotronic weapons." In this report they defined psychotronics as the " the projection or transmission of mental energy by individual or collective mental discipline and control, or by an energy-emitting device-a kind of jammer." This report then stated definitively that the technology, physics, and mathematics involved are real, and not matter of the occult or anything supernatural. While this may seem somewhat hard to believe, apprehensions concerning international advances in psychotronic weaponry has reached extremes among a number of primarily retired U.S. military officials.

Even as recently as 1987, the U.S. Army considered how psychokinesis could be used as a means of disturbing enemy computer systems, triggering nuclear weapons, for even destroying weapons and vehicles. I do believe that the energy we call PK is connected to the supernatural, while these materialistic scientists do not concur. J.B. Rhine the main pioneer of institutional PK research believed that it is a gross error to treat psychokinesis as a physical force. He knew good and well that is an aspect of the will, soul and of consciousness which are not bound to the limitations of physical laws.

Obviously there are many different theories about how PK works, but good physicists and enlightened ones know that ultimately we are dealing with some of illusion (Maya) controlled by certain energetic principles. The yogic doctrines teach that the energy is an important part of controlling the material nature and life itself. Leading scientists such as Helmut Schmidt have began making the most powerful PK breakthroughs only through the precepts of quantum physics. That whole body of knowledge is based on micro-level illusion.

In the end, quantum physics pertains to controlling the very same illusion that the world scriptures have told us about since very remote times. Even in remote Vedic times, there were telekinetic weapons that functioned at a subatomic level, such as the *Bramastra* revealed to us in the *Srimad Bhagavatam*. According to *Srimad Bhagavatam* in the *First Canto*, the Bramastra weapon was used more than 5,000 years ago in Battle, as an engineered mantric cocktail that was apparently more powerful and precise than atomic weapons of today. It was apparently designed to work on a quantum level and telekinetic power was a major aspect of this weapon. The main concern regarding these kinds of threats including atomic warfare is how we can protect ourselves from them.

Queen Kunti, a great devotee of Lord Sri Krsna had a son named emperor Majaraja Praksit. He became the emperor of the entire planet 5,000 years ago following the battle of Kuruksetra. This was a major historical battle presented in the *Mahabharata*, where people fought from all parts of the world. This was the battlefield in India where Lord Sri Krsna spoke the entire *Bhagavad-Gita* to His disciple Arjuna just prior to combat. The *Mahabharata* is one of the greatest spiritual epics of all times and is a powerful tool for transcendentalism.

The psychokinetic bramastra weapon was used on emperor Praksit when he was still in his mother Uttara's womb. According to Srila Prabhupada, the bramastra weapon was even more powerful and precise than nuclear weapons of today. Prabhupada said, "another advantage of this weapon is that it is not blind like the nuclear weapon because it can be directed only to the target and nothing else." The scriptures report that the emperor's mother, Uttara, knew the weapon had been used on her. *Srimad Bhagavatam* says that the emperor felt the heat while he was in the belly. By the way this also indicates that a fetus can sense and feel. Due to the extreme power of the bramastra weapon, there was no hope outside of Lord Sri Krsna for their survival.

The advanced telekinetic brahmastra weapon generated radiation similar to that created by atomic weaponry of today. Still, this was no threat for the Hand of God. When Uttara knew that the psychokinetic weapon was used against her, she began to pray for Lord Sri Krsna's divine protection. The Lord easily foiled the force used against His devotee and the emperor survived the attack, while in his mother's womb. Lord Krnsa used His all powerful Sudarsana Disk to destroy the most highly advanced psychokinetic weapon, just for protecting His devotees who were surrendered. These short excerpts from Srimad Bhagavatam illustrate the power of the Lord's

Hand in protecting His devotees:

SB 1.8.13:

" *The almighty Personality of Godhead, Sri Krsna, having observed that a great danger was befalling His unalloyed devotees, who were fully surrendered souls, at once took up His Sudarsana disk to protect them.*"

S.B. 1.8.15:

"*Although the Supreme Bramastra weapon released by Asvatthama was irresistible and without check or counteraction, it was neutralized when confronted by the strength of Vishnu [Lord Krsna].*"

S.B. 1.8.17:

"*Thus saved from the radiation of the bramastra, Kunti, the chaste devotee of the Lord, and her five sons and Draupadi addressed Lord Krsna as He started for home.*"

Many scientists in modern times are increasingly concerned with the threats posed by PK weaponry. As you have seen thought this manuscript, I have discovered that Lord Sri Krsna is a direct connection to supreme that well of telekinetic power. Prayer for Krsna's divine protection, and surrendering unto Him is the best shield against all hurt, harm and danger! With nations persisting in threats of nuclear warfare and related weapons development, surrendering to Krsna is the most intelligent way to protect yourself. He directly tells us in the *Bhagavad-Gita* that " I am smaller than the smallest particle." This means that Lord Sri Krsna can work on the most minute sub-atomic levels to shield His devotees from all peril.

In response to the growing concerns about psychokinetic weapons programs abroad, The United States Psychotronics Association was established by retired US military official Tom Bearden. He argues that PK weapons programs abroad present very serious apocalyptic threats. He claimed to have secret inside information that certain nations have developed highly effective PK weaponry. In fact, many people maintain that a US submarine ship called the USS Thresher was destroyed by the Soviets in 1964 experiment involving a psychotronics military weapon. It was the deadliest submarine disaster in history. Bearden and a host of others believe that Russia developed a weapon in the 1960's, which uses "time-polarized EM waves" to disrupt the normal flow of time, and used that it was used in Afghanistan during the 1980s.

Bearden has also claimed that Russia used various other technologies in the 1980's to cause the destruction of the Challenger space shuttle and induce "several large earthquakes." The mysterious destruction of the atom submarine was a major disaster where 129 people were lost in waters 220 miles of the Boston coast. While some scientist are skeptical about Bearden's views, many others confirmed the existence of psychotronics and PK in general. One US military report stated, "the technology, physics, and mathematics involved with PK developments are unequivocally real and not a matter of occult fiction." A growing number of scientists believe that potential military purposes and applications of PK force include the hindering of nuclear weapons, fighting aircraft, and producing disruptive weather conditions.

After many years of research in the area, the advancement of telekinetic weaponry still remains an unsolved mystery, due to the secrecy of military developments. In light of all of the research, no material scientist can account for what causes PK or its origins within the context of contemporary science or physics. Many scientists accept the position of J.B. Rhine regarding PK force--that is "a product of the higher mind and the soul." Of course, scientific breakthroughs in the field of PK are not limited to weapons development applications. Many researchers are exploring biological applications of PK energy, and they hypothesize that it may lead to control over genetics and maybe even evolution. Many others are principally concerned with how this force can be used to manifest our deepest hopes and dreams.

It is believed by many researchers in the field that this force can actually be generated and transmitted. In fact, Soviets have long encouraged the exploration of a relationship between technology and PK. Interestingly, the FP specifically relates to that field of interest–modern technology and PK. The research in PK is predicted to follow two paths: The first is to pursue techniques for improving a person's psychic ability to direct PK or ESP more precisely and effectively at a specific target. The other is to devise *some system* in which a known type of energy (i.e. prana or life-force) is used to amplify anybody's relatively weak PK potential.

Of course, our interests, intents and purposes are concerned solely with using these technologies for self help, spiritual advancement and personal achievement. Please note that the psychotronic technologies I endorse have powerful effects on enhancing physical and spiritual yoga along with any other metaphysical and occult practices. There are now quite effective psychotronic technologies available, which were invented by various enlightened and progressive bio-physicists. These machines can be used to amplify anybody's natural telekinetic mind over matter powers. I have used telekinetic devices for personal and spiritual development for many years. I personally confirm the effectiveness and extreme power in using these technologies.

One example of such a device is a small machine that charges (loads) water with prana energy, which triggers a substantial boost in one's natural PK levels. In fact, many people, myself included, can literally feel a massive energetic boost all over the body as soon as this "charged water" even touches our lips. Many people have developed the opinion that this application of using of psychotronic energy can have certain holistic health benefits. Again, prana is one of the most instantly effective PK triggers and I have proved it repeatedly. Essentially, the more of this charged water that one drinks, the more psychic, telekinetic and spiritual power one develops. Interestingly enough, I drank plenty of charged Shakti water right before the greatest spiritual awakenings began happening in my life!

Another kind of psychotronics device I have used is a small prana energy generator that plugs right into the wall. It projects an energy field into the environment, or where ever the operator intends. These devices naturally and immediately boosts the levels of telekinetic powers in the environment. It throws important bio-energetic spiritual processes into motion. In terms of the FP, I have personally conducted controlled experiments using this kind of machine, and the results are shocking. As you have read, I have actually "jump started" my refrigerator with one device. I have also shut the fridge down in my home and replicated this feat in the homes of disciples. Again, this is all accounted for within the ancient principles of Mahayana Buddhism that we have already explored many times in this handbook.

I can certainly confirm that this kind of mind over matter apparatus is highly effective for empowering the mind to control matter on all levels. These machines definitely produce prana energy which in turn boosts the ultimate energy Kundalini. Many people believe that Prana energy can not be produced which is untrue. It has been proven that this life energy can be controlled and harnessed by Western scientists such as Reich and Mesmer. The next logical step in human evolution is the ability to produce it. Some say that because Prana is everywhere, it can not be produced. My response is that although prana is everywhere, it still must be filtered from the air. One must know how to do this by using prescribed yogic methods. Certain technologies work with the natural laws to produce life force and control it. Before electricity could be produced, it was also observed, studied, harnessed and controlled. Scientists had first to realize that magnetic fields effect the electric charge of coils and that the coils also produced magnetic fields, before they could proceed to invent the electric generator. Psychotronics gadgets tremendously amplify PK abilities and psi performance. In a technological age driven by frequencies and atomic physics, it is certainly beneficial to use these most cutting edge technologies. Since we use technology in virtually every other area of our lives, it makes sense to extend this pattern into our mental and spiritual development. If God was fundamentally opposed to technology, then He would not permit the whole world to rest upon it.

There is an unequivocal and direct connection between my supernatural powers, the functioning of refrigerators of all kinds, and the use of cutting edge psychotronic technology. You can find more detailed information about these types of psychotronics developments at www.thisispk.org. For me, it only takes small bursts of PK energy from a PK amp to jump start a fridge or shut it down. There appears to be a direct connection between the functioning of matter as a whole and the use of PK amplifiers. Therefore, I encourage you all to experiment carefully with these devices, and then draw your own conclusions about how they work best. One thing for certain is that they do create a massive boost in one's ability to control material phenomenon. The only way to find out how telekinetic you really are is to run a test with the psychotronic triggers and energy generators. I encourage everybody interested in the realities of mind over matter to at least experiment and run one test with a psychotronics device.

In working with psychotronics, it is crucial to note that it usually takes time to work. The amount of time that it takes to manifest and materialize something can vary tremendously. The main to remember is that nature has to take its course. Everything in nature is bound by time. The big picture concept is described in the Gita–that by its very nature, the mind controls matter and is a superior form of energy. Since everything including man animals and planty life comes directly from nature the power to control it is ineffable. Earth, air, fire, water, and ether are all elements that magicians over time have found helps the mind to control nature within the context of "magick." What we consider to be magical is really only scientific. It is interesting how the FP discovery relates specifically to both science and mysticism or religion. Psychotronics also captures the essence of both scientific and religious thought. Perhaps that accounts for its extreme power and effectiveness

Although magick and psi are not not the same, magick works on the power of psi, mind power, and its inherent ability to control matter and nature. Along the same lines, psychotronics that is backed with life energy (prana) not only amplifies anybody's PK abilities, it naturally loosens the slack between the mind and matter. That empowers the mind to control it more effectively. I think that also accounts for why these life energy boosted psychotronics technologies tend to help most people sleep much better. According to my Austrian Guru, Sri Pranananda who is an expert in *hatha-yoga* and generating life energy, "life energy makes any technology work much better." The human body is nothing more than a technology, which is why it is also associated with healing, growth and fertility. When we conceive of life itself as one huge technology, then we see the big picture. Life force and the resulting PK power somehow makes this technology called life work much better under the control of the mind and thoughts!

I have certainly made important breakthroughs in life and in understanding mind over matter by daily use of these machines. I truly believe that they can change anybody's life, by giving them powerful mind over matter experiences that they can control. It is only God that blesses us with tools like these that can be used to improve our lives and karma. Psychotronic mind machines have unquestionably played a major part in changing my entire life for the better, by triggering the hidden divine forces within. Why is this the case? Well, its plainly and simply because the mind is so accustomed to using technology for everything from driving to eating. So when we tune into technology for spiritual purposes, it is much easier for the mind to function on that level. I have been astounded by the results of using them in daily life and for experimental purposes. I endorse these technologies to my growing base of disciples and fellow devotees around the world. Many experienced physicists and other professionals agree that these devices are incredibly effective. With practice and experimentation, anybody can develop strong and reliable telekinetic powers that can be used for any purpose desired.

It is always quite entertaining to observe PK practitioners such as

Uri Geller in action bending forks and spoons on stage! However, we should focus on how this cosmic force can be used to literally *bend life itself* in the right direction! Stage entertainment is always fun and healthy, but on a more serious note, as yogis mastering the science of life, we want to understand, enhance, and control this energy. Those that remain mentally "entertained," captivated by material energies and miracles can never control them without a deeper understanding.

Intensive study of how PK works enables one to achieve success known as "psi hits" consistently in one's psychotronics operations. It is clear based on the evidence of psi research that with enough attempts, nearly anybody can eventually achieve a psi hit. That is why the element of persistence in any undertaking is essential for success. When the mind's power is intensively focused on something, it definitely can affect it. So, we need to use this secret knowledge to manifest when we want and need for this life and the next.   That is very crucial to note because it implies that we can create anything we want in our lives using these tools and technologies that God has introduced us to. Of course, the main purpose of any psychotronics action is to achieve a "psi hit" instead of a "psi miss." Therefore, we need to understand how to increase the odds of success in any psychotronics operation.

 I have discovered that by working through the chakras using the methods and processes described in this handbook, we can greatly increase control over matter and success in psychotronics operations. For example, chanting certain mystical mantras causes the energy to rise to the heart chakra. As a natural result, more creative power resonates within the throat chakra, as it naturally drifts upward. This makes it much easier to succeed in your psychotronic mind over matter operations because the throat chakra is your center of creativity. Other mantras cause the life energy to resonate specifically in the throat chakra which gives more creative powers in your psychotronics work. Similarly, it is quite effective to work within the realm of the solar plexus chakrs, which is the seat of will power. Simply tune into that chakra using one of many methods, and then perform the psychotronics operation specifically willing for your desire to manifest. All of this advise is here to help make your life much easier, which is the same reason why we use any form of technology. In terms of becoming perpetually telekinetic, learning to use a psychotronics devise is one of the best methods.

Many researchers have also found that entering into certain altered states of consciousness can boost PK performance and psi hitting. For example, Charles Honorton found that a practitioner of transcendental meditation scored significantly higher for half of his trials, after he performed certain meditation (but not before or during). A similar follow up study involving practitioners of *Ajapa-yoga* reported psi-missing prior to meditation, but not during or after. Like any field of science or research, by analyzing which variables affect the big picture, we learn a whole lot about how to control it.

In another study, there were two groups: Of course, an experimental and control groups, where 25 members of the experimental group practiced some form of transcendental meditation before the experiment, and 25 control subjects did not. The difference in the two groups was significant. The experimental group scored significantly better than chance. On the other hand, the control groups scored below chance expectation.

The results of these studies certainly indicate that yoga, transcendental meditation, and inducing altered states of consciousness is a variable that is perhaps determinative of success or failures in all mind over matter or psychotronics endeavors. It is no surprise in light of these studies that I stumbled upon the FP while engaged in some form of transcendental yoga (japa meditation). Shakti work and chakra yoga are definitely other forms of transcendental meditation that give us more direct mind over matter control. Again, chakra meditation, clearing and development prior to performing a psychotronics operation is very powerful for boosting success.

Psychotronics is kind of like of a game, where you either hit or miss, depending on a lot of variables. The secret is to recognize what variables need to be manipulated in your mind to achieve a success in your psychotronics operations. In that respect, these technologies bring lots of fun into life, especially when we realize that life is nothing but a really long dream and an illusion. These exciting technologies are engineered to help us control the illusion for any purpose desired. However, we must not forget that the ultimate psi-hit miracle is using our mind over matter skills and technologies to make it back to the Kingdom of God, after we depart the Earth.

You can have as much fun as you like using psychotronics developments, but it can never compare to the fun and perfection experienced in the Lord's Supreme abode. This special place is reserved for the highest yogis. In the material world, we are all so limited by space and time in our capacity to enjoy anything. No matter how much bread we have, there is only so much space in our belly to accommodate it. No matter how much fun there is to have, there is only so much time in the material world before its all over! That is why I urge readers to seek the face of God for the highest pleasure. And, to use your power, technology and intelligence to please Him.

My advanced telekinetic powers are a direct result of deep meditation and introspection, God-consciousness and disciplinary yoga. I have mastered this energy in such as way that I can do more with it then merely entertain people. I am in the business of helping people to help themselves with this divine force. That is a main dichotomy between myself and other world famous PK practitioners. Although many telekinetic people have been studied so closely in the laboratories, we still must wonder what this all has produced, in terms of practical useful solutions and direction for our lives! What spiritual value does such staged entertainment have?

Even if one person can perform endless miracles and feats, the whole point is lost if one can not teach others to exploit this same force. That is because there is only so much time to enjoy any given feat. Thus we should not be sidetracked by miracles, but instead we should use them to understand our true nature and existence.

People are trying so hard to understand this force towards the degree that PK research is now the fastest growing field of parapsychology. On the other hand, there are yogis, sages and transcendentalists who know that The Lord is smaller than the smallest particle and all powerful. These devotees can understand, control and direct this same force with ease! Moreover, within transcendental science, the progress has been made long ago in terms of how this energy can be used.

Although many mainstream researchers claim this is an energy with no spiritual basis or origins, I adamantly dissent. If they know so much about this energy, why are they unable to use it, help others with it, enhance it or even understand it after more than 100 years in the laboratory? By the way, I did not discover the FP during a laboratory research trial or while studying a science course book under the false impression that divine telekinetic energy is bound to those conditions. I was engaged in transcendental and loving devotional service unto God when I discovered this psychic phenomenon. When God is pleased with our service unto Him, then He gives us power over these divine energies, and profound enlightenment comes along with that. I think that mystical experiences and subsequent enlightenment is the greatest gift of all aside from Love of God.

I have found the solutions to all of my problems through working closely with this divine energy. My own life has demonstrated how effective that PK energy and its techno-triggers can be in terms producing real miracles consistently; and for totally improving life for anybody who is open minded. I have given you the keys to success, for the rest of your entire life! Recall again that this energy acts independently of us, and we must only learn to summon it, or simply call it up, by raising its levels, by using integrated and innovative PK triggers and psychotronic technology.

In a time on Earth marked by unprecedented change, people should unite to raise this energy for using it in ways that are productive and regenerating. The key issue is how our PK can be used in ways that benefit us all, and vanquish all manners of suffering; to purify the planet, create heavenly conditions right here and to combat evil, darkness and destructive forces. This Shakti Sankirtana Movement is about leading all who desire to the highest standards of living.

This divine energy has compelled me to teach people all over the world how to overcome any predicaments, persecution, tribulations, *personal injuries*, setbacks and spirtual issues. The unlimited powers of God and His sacred technologies can do anything for those who learn to work with it. Sacred psychotronic technologies are only available through the grace of Lord Sri Krsna, who is the Supreme Yogi. It is only the Hand of God that opened this channel for learning how to control this energy, for creating whatever we want in life; and to solve all of our problems if we will only believe.

Here, you have been given the information, tools, knowledge and sheer power to write your own ticket; and, to change every dimension of your life for the better by using PK force. Evidently, your personal karma has empowered you to evolve on the cutting-edge, instead of being left behind, and out in the cold, without any specialized information about psychotronics. Since the divine PK force can bring you anything you will for in life, it is your responsibility is to aim high. As a human being, you should know how to avoid the greatest miseries through the power of higher mind. In this material world, there are always competing forces of positive and negative energies. That is particularly true or this age of Kali.

The secret of life is to tune the mind in totally on the positive frequencies. When we focus the mind on the positive things in our lives, then everything becomes positive, which is a natural mind over matter effect. The most positive thing that one can ever think of is Lord Sri Krsna Himself. Incidentally, He instructs us in the Gita to "Just always think of Me." Since even the most agitated mind can naturally rest at its best while absorbed in Krsna, transcendental meditation on Him, as an actual person, is the key to restoring peace, opulence and prosperity in our lives.

By constantly engaging the mind in thinking of Sri Krsna and His pastimes, our individual souls are dovetailed with the Supreme soul.

That accounts for the major increases in telekinesis and other mystic psi phenomenon resulting from transcendental practices such as *bhakti-yoga*. All of this fosters positive permanent karmic change in our lives which is absolutely critical! This information is certainly invaluable for those who are willing to concede that things have not been working under the status quo for much of this planet, and that it is time to try something new. As soon as you think it you are there! So, by merely thinking of Sri Krsna who is undeniably divine, you become one with Him in yoga.

Moreover, His sublime power halts all negative influences and destructive forces in our environments. On the other hand, His divine energy (Hara) opens the chakras up to the receive the positive frequencies. The divine power of Krsna is so potent that it naturally banishes all evil, which makes it possible for us to become thoroughly successful and happy. Whenever one senses peril or evil in any world where the mind goes, one can simple chant the Holy Names of God and it will definitely go away. As the heart is gradually purified by fixing the mind of God as a *transcendental person*, the soul is naturally elevated to the highest planetary systems. In fact, Lord Sri Krsna confirms in the Gita that those who conceptualize of the Supreme as a person, and meditate on Him in that form, are the highest yogis. He's just a person that lives on a different planet; the highest planet in the spiritual world (Krsnaloka). He is not an ordinary person, as He is *transcendental*, all knowing, all-powerful, and the Supreme Controller of everything that be. The FP discovery, which directly resulted from the practice of *bhakti-yoga,* has opened the door for anybody to see the Supreme Absolute Truth for what it really is.

Bibliography

1.Stanley Krippner, *Advances in Parapsychological Research: Vol.1: Psychokinesis.* Springer;1 edition (November 1, 1977)
2. Bacon, F. *The New Atlantis.* Chicago: Encyclopedia Britannica, 1952. (Originally published, 1627)
3. Bailey, Alice, the yoga Sutras of Patanjali, Lucis Publishing House, New York, 1949.
4. Barry, J. General and comparative study of the psychokinetic

effects on a fungus culture. Journal of Parapsychology, 1968, 32, 237-243.

5. Barry, Jean. "General and Comparative Study of the Psychokinetic Effect on a Fungus Culture." Journal of Parapsychology 32 (1968):237-43.

6. Behanan, K.T. *Yoga: A Scientific Evaluation*, Macmillan, New York, 1937.

7. Bender, H. The case of "Silvio" and some others. In J.D. Morris, W.G. Roll, and R.L. Morris (Eds.), Research in parapsychology 1976. Metuchen, N.J.: Scarecrow Press, 1977, in press.

8. Bender, H., Vandrey, R., and Wendlandt, S. The "Geller effetc" in Western Germany and Switzerland: A preliminary report on a social and experimental study. In J. D. Morris, W. G. Roll, and R.L Morris (Eds.), Research in parapsychology 1975. Metuchen, N.J.: Scarecrow Press, 1976, 141-144.

9.Andrija Puharich, *Beyond Telepathy*. Doubleday & Co., Inc.

10.Brier, R.M. PK on a bio-electric system. Journal of Parapsychology, 1969, 33, 187-205.

11.Ambika Wauters. *The Book of Chakras*. Barron's, 2002.

12.Butler, J.A. V., Electrical Phenomenon at Interfaces, Methuen, London, 1951, p.265.

13.Carrel, Alexis. *The Voyage to Lourdes*. New York: Harper & Brothers, 1950.

14.Blawyn and Jones. *Chakra Workout for Body, Mind and Spirit*. Llewellyn Publications, 1993.

15.Charles Johnson. *The Yoga Sutras of Patanjali*. London, 1949.

16.Chauvin, R., and Genthon, P.P. An investigation of the possibility of PK experiments with uranium and a Geiger counter. Journal of Parapsychology, 1967, 31, 168. (Abstract)

17.Cox, W.E. Note on some experiments with Uri Geller. Journal of Parapsychology, 1974, 38, 408-411.

18.Cox, W.E. Blind PK with automated equipment. Journal of Parapsychology, 1976, 40, 48. (Abstract)

19.Crookes, W. Researches in the phenomenon of spiritualism. London: J. Burns, 1874

20.Crookes, Sir William, Researchers in Spiritualism, pp 34-42

21.David-Neel, op. cit. W.Y. Evans-Wentz, Tibet's Great Yoga Milarepa

22.Dunraven, Earl of (Lord Adare). Experiences in Spiritualism with D.D. Home: Society for Psychical Research

23.Eisenbud, J. The world of Ted Serios. New York: William Morrow, 1967.

24.Forwald, H. Mind, matter, and gravitation: A theoretical and experimental study (Parapsychological monographs No. 11). New York: Parapsychology Foundation, 1969.

25. Franklin, W. Fracture surface physics indicating teleneural interaction. New Horizons, 1975, 2(1), 8-13

26. I.K. Taimni, Glimpses into the Psychology of Yoga, The Theosophical Publishing House, 1976.

27. Grad, B.A telekinetic effect on plant growth. International Journal of Parapsychology, 1963, 5(2),117-133.

28.Grad, B.A telekinetic effect on plant growth, II. Experiments involving treatment of saline in stoppered bottles. International Journal of Parapsychology, 1964, 6(4), 473-498.

29.Grad, B. A telekinetic effect on yeast activity. Journal of Parapsychology, 1965, 29, 285-186.

30.Grad, Bernard. "The Biological Effects of the Laying on of Hands" on Animals and Plants: Implications for Biology," in G. Schmeidler (ed.), Parapsychology: Its Relation to Physics, Biology, Psychology and Psychiatry. Metuchen, N.J.:Scarecrow Press, 1976.

31.Green, E. Report to the Third Interdisciplinary Conference on the Voluntary Control of Internal States, Council Grove, Kansas, 1971.

32.Haraldsson, E. Psychokinetic effects on yeast: An exploration experiment. In W.G. Roll, R.L. Morris, and J.D. Morris (Eds.), Research in Parapsychology 1972. Metuchen, N.J.: Scarecrow Press, 1973, 20-21.

33.Hasted, J.B. An experimental study of the validity of the metal bending phenomena. Journal of the Society for Psychical Research, 1976, 48, 365-383.

34. Hill, S."PK Effects by a Single Subject on a Binary Random Number Generator Based on Electric Noise," in Research in Parapsychology 1976, J.D. Morris, W.G. Roll, and R.L. Morris, eds. (Metuchen, N.J.: The Scarecro Press, 1977), pp. 26-28.

35. His Divine Grace A.C. Bhaktivedanta Swami Prabhupada. *Sri Isopanistad*, The Bhaktivedanta Book Trust, 1969.

36. His Divine Grace A.C. Bhaktivedanta Swami Prabhupada, *Bhagavad-Gita As it is*, Bhaktivedanta Book Trust, 1989.

37. His Divine Grace A.C. Bhaktivedanta Swami Prabhupada. *Krsna The Supreme Personality of Godhead*. The Bhaktivedanta Book Trust,1972.

38. Honorton, C. Apparent psychokinesis on static objects by a "gifted" subject. In W. G. Roll, R.L. Morris, and J.D Morris (Eds.), Research in parapsychology 1973. Metuchen, N.J.: Scarecrow Press, 1974, pp. 128-131.

39. Honorton, C. Effects of Meditation and feedback on psychokinetic performance: A pilot study with an instructor of TM (Transcendental Meditation). In J.D. Morris, W.G. Roll, and R.L. Morris (Eds.), Research in Parapsychology 1976, Metuchen, N.J.: Scarecrow Press, 1977, in press.

40.Honorton, C. "Has Science Developed the Competence to Confront Claims of the Paranormal?" Presidential Address, P.A. Convention, August 1975, in Research in Parapsychology 1975, J.D. Morris, W. G. Roll, and R.L. Morris, eds. (Metuchen, N.J.: The Scarecrow Press, 1976),pp.19-223.parapsychology 26(1965):140-147.

41.Honorton, C., & Krippner, S. Hypnosis and ESP performance. Journal of the American Society for Psychical Research. 1969, 63, 214-252

42.Honorton, C. Psi-conducive states of awareness, In E.D. Mitchell and others, Psychic exploration: A challenge for science. New York: Putnam's, 1974.

43.Keil, H.H.J., Herbert, B., Ullman, M., and Pratt. J.G. Directly observable voluntary PK effects. Proceedings of the Society for Psychical Research, 1976, 56, 197-235

44. Swami Muktananda. *Kundalini The Secret of Life*. SYDA Foundation, 1978.

45. Khalsa, K. Shakta. *Kundalini Yoga*. New York, New York: A Penguin Company, 2001.

46.Mann, W. Edward. Orgone, Reich and Eros. New York: Simon & Schuster, 1973.

47. Matas, F., and Pantas, L.A PK experiment comparing meditation versus nonmeditation subjects. In W.G. Roll, R.L. Morris, and J.D. Morris (Eds.), Proceedings of Parapsychological Association No. 8, 1971. Durham, N.C.: Parapsychological Association, 1972, 12-13.

48. Matsunaga, Alicia. The Buddhist Philosophy of Assimilation. Rutland, Vt.: Charles E. Tuttle Co., 1969.

49. May, E.C., and Honorton, C. A dynamic PK experiment with Indigo Swann. In J.D. Morris, W.G. Roll, and R.L. Morris (Eds.), Research in parapsychology 1975. Metuchen, N.J.:Scarecrow Press, 1976, pp. 88-89

50. *Minds and Motion: The Riddle of Psychokinesis.* Taplinger Publishing Co, Inc. First Edition (1978).

51. Nash, C.B., and Nash, C.S. Effect of paranormally conditioned solution on yeast fermentation. Journal of Parapsychology, 1967, 31, 314. (Abstract)

52. Osty, E., and Osty, M. Les Pouvoirs inconnus de l'espirit sur la matiere. Revue Metapsychique, 1931, No. 6, 393-427, and 1932, No. 1, 1-59

53. Owen, A. R. G. Uri Geller's metal phenomena: an eyewitness account. New Horizons, 1974, 1(4), 164-171.(b)

54. Owen, I.M. "Phillip's" story continued. New Horizons, 1975, 2(1), 14-20.

55. Parker, A. States of Mind: ESP and altered states of consciousness. New York: Taplinger, 1975.

56. Panati, C. The Geller papers. Boston: Houghton-Mifflin, 1976

57. Pauli, E. N. El poder de la mente sobre objectivos vivientes. Cuadernos de Parapsicologia, 1974, 7, 1-14.

58. Pratt, J.G. The Cormack Placement PK Experiments. Journal of Parapsychology, 1951,15, 57-73.

59. Price, H. Rudi Schneider: A scientific examination of his mediumship. London: Methuen, 1930.

60. Price, H. Stella C.: An account of some original experiments in psychical research. London: Souvenir Press, 1973. (Originally published, 1925.)

61. Puthoff, H., and Targ, R. PK experiments with Uri Geller and Indigo Swann. In W.G. Roll, R.L. Morris, and J.D. morriss (Eds.), Research in parapsychology 1973

62. Puthoff, H., and Targ, R. Psychic research and modern physics. In E.D. Mitchell, and others. Psychic exploration: A challenge for science. New York: Putnam's, 1974.

63. Puthoff, H., and Targ, R. Psychic research and modern physics. In E.D. Mitchell, and others. Psychic exploration: A challenge for science. New York: Putnam's, 1974.

64. Puthoff, H., and Targ, R. Physics, entropy, and psychokinesis. In Laura Oteri (Ed.), Quantum physics and parapsychology. New York: Parapsychology Foundation, 1975.

65. Raknes, Ola. Wilhelm Reich and orgonomy. Baltimore: Pelican Books, 1970.

66. Rhine, L.E. ESP in life and lab: Tracing hidden channels. New York: Macmillan, 1967.

67. Rhine, L.E. Placement PK tests with three types of objects. Journal of Parapsychology, 1951.

68. Richet, C. Thirty years of psychical research. New York: Macmillan, 1923

69. Richmond, Nigel. "Two Series of PK Tests on Paramecia." Jounral of the Society for Psychical Research 36 (1956):577-88.

70 Rose, L. Faith Healing. Baltimore, Md, Penguin Books, 1971.

71. His Divine Grace A.C. Bhaktivedanta Swami Prabhupada, *Srimad Bhagavatam First Canto: Creation."* The Bhaktivedanta Book Trust, 1985.

72. Schmeidler, G. R. PK effects upon continuously recorded temperature. Journal of the American Society for Psychical Research, 1973, 67, 325-340.

73. Schmidt, H. A PK test with electronic equipment. Journal of Parapsychology, 1970, 34, 175-181.(a)

74. Schmidt, H., and Pantas, L. Psi tests with internally fifferent machines. Journal of Parapsychology, 1972, 36, 222-232.

75. Schmidt, H. Precognition of a quantum process. Journal of Parapsychology, 1969, 33, 99-108.

76. Schmidt, H. "Instrumentation in the Parapsychology

Laboratory," in New Directions in Parapsychology, J. Beloff, ed. (Metuchen, N.J: The Scarecrow Press, 1975), pp.13-37.
77. Simonton, Carl. "The Role of the Mind in Cancer Therapy," in Stanley Dean (ed.), {pssychiatry and Mysticism. Chicago: Nelson-Hall, 1975.
78. Smith, M.J. Paranormal effects on enzyme activity. Human Dimensions, 1972, 1(2), 15-19.
79. Smith Justa. "Paranormal Effect of Enzyme Activity Through Laying-On-of-hands," Human Dimensions, Summer 1972.
80. Stevenson, I., and Pratt, J.G. Exploratory investigations of the psychic photography of Ted Serios. Journal of the American Society for Psychical Research, 1968, 62, 103-129.
81.The yoga Sutras of Patanjali, Tr. by Rama Prasad, Sudhindranath Vasu, Allahabad, 1924.
82.Master Subramuniya. *The Book of Affirmations*. Fourth edition. Comstock House, 1973
83. Jean Houston. *The Possible Human*. Houghton Mifflin Company, 1982.
84.Paramahansa Yogananda. *Autobiography of a Yogi*. Rider& Co, 1946..
85.Barrie R. Cassileth, Ph.D., W.W. Norton & Co.,The Alternative Medicine. Handbook,1998
86. Diana Robinson, *To Stretch a Plank: A Survey of Psychokinesis*. Burnham Inc., June 1989.
87. Watkins, G.K., and Watkins, A.M. Apparent psychokinesis on static objects by a "gifted" subject: A laboratory demonstration . In W.G. Roll, R.L. Morris, and J.D. Morris (Eds.), Research in parapsychology 1973. Metuchen, N.J.: Scarecrow Press, 1974, pp. 125-128.
88.Worrall, A., and Worrall, O. The gift of healing. New York: Harper & Rowe, 1965.
89.Watkins, G., and Watkins, A. "Possible PK Influences on the Resuscitation of Anesthetized Mice." 99. Journal of Parapsychology 35(1971):257-72.
90. West, D.J. Eleven Lourdes Miracles. New York: Garrett Publications, 1957.
91.W.Y. Evans-Wentz, The Tibetan Book of Great Liberation, or the Method of Realizing Nirvana through Knowing the Mind, Oxford, 1951.
92. W.Y. Evans-Wentz. *Tibetan Yoga and Secret Doctrines*. Oxford, 1935.
93. Winnett, R., and Hornorton, C. Effects of Meditation and feedback on psychokinetic performance: Results with practitioners of Ajapa yoga. In J.D. Morris, W.G. Roll, and R.l. Morris (Eds.), Research in parapsychology 1976. Metuchen, N.J.: Scarecrow Press, 1977, in press.
94) Hill, Napolian. *Think and Grow Rich*. Hawthorne Books Inc, 1968

Printed in the United States
131647LV00001B/186/P

9 780615 237374